1 MO1
FREE
READING

at
www.ForgottenBooks.com

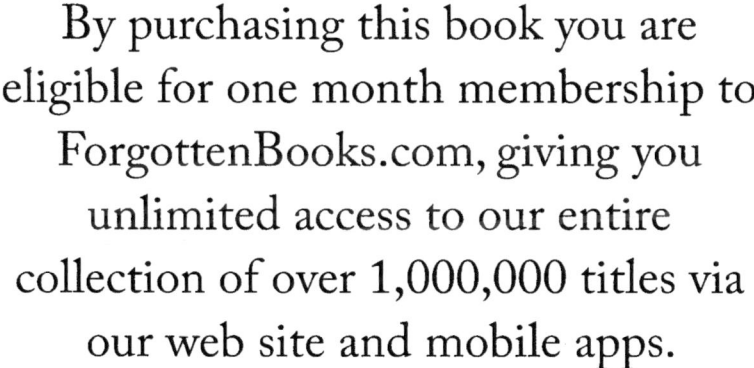

By purchasing this book you are eligible for one month membership to ForgottenBooks.com, giving you unlimited access to our entire collection of over 1,000,000 titles via our web site and mobile apps.

To claim your free month visit:

www.forgottenbooks.com/free871719

MW01609065

ISBN 978-0-266-58924-2
PIBN 10871719

PREFACE.

THE following pages are intended as a concise practical guide by which the general public may become familiar with the causes, symptoms, prevention, and treatment, of the more common diseases that may be successfully treated at home.

The manual will be found to contain much valnable information for every family and individual; and frequent reference to it will, in many cases, save the necessity of consulting a physician and paying large consultation fees.

If you desire to keep well, you can learn how to do it from these pages; if you would keep your children well, follow the advice herein given; if you are sick, consult this manual and you will know what to do at once. In short, you will find this work an ever-ready medical adviser, upon which you can rely as certainly as if you consulted the most experienced specialist in any of the diseases described.

It covers all the subjects that are contained in the large and expensive works on Domestic Medicine, in such condensed form that all information sought for can be obtained in a few moments.

The treatment recommended and the directions given for preserving health are the most approved and scientific of the present day, and the work is in every way up to date, while all the older works on popular medicine are from fifteen to thirty years behind the age.

The medicines recommended are such as are used by the leading physicians of America and Europe, and all prescriptions are given in plain terms that can be understood by every reader.

The symptoms of many surgical diseases are described, so that they can be readily recognized before serious deformities result, thus enabling the sufferer to consult a surgeon in time to insure a radical cure of the trouble, and thus save much unnecessary suffering.

Our first aim is to teach people how to preserve health and prevent disease; while, to those who are already victims of the sequences of violated laws, we offer the most approved remedies and the best advice for the restoration of health.

A perusal of these pages will convince every reader of the importance of complying with the old axiom, " Know thyself;" and those who follow the rules and advice herein contained will demonstrate for themselves the great good that can be derived by instructing the people regarding the nature and treatment of the diseases to which they are liable.

R. A. GUNN, M. D.,
Consulting Physician and Surgeon.

CONTENTS.

CHAPTER I.

THE ORGANS OF DIGESTION.

How to Preserve Health—Diseases of the Digestive Organs—Acute Indigestion—Chronic Dyspepsia—Catarrh of the Stomach—Jaundice— Diarrhea— Chronic Diarrhea— Cholera Morbus—Dysentery—Cholera Infantum —Habitual Constipation—Worms.......... 13

CHAPTER II.

MALARIAL DISEASES.

Malarial Fevers — Intermittent Fever — Remittent, or Bilious, Fever.................... 38

CHAPTER III.

SPECIFIC GERM DISEASES.

Small-Pox—Chicken-Pox — Measels—Erysipelas —Cholera—Yellow Fever—Diphtheria—La Grippe, or Influenza—Hay Fever—Whooping Cough—Mumps—Typhoid Fever...... 43

CHAPTER IV.

DISEASES OF DEFECTIVE NUTRITIAN.

Rheumatism—Gout—Diabetes—Rickets—Scrof-
ula. 64

CHAPTER V.

SPECIFIC BLOOD DISEASES.

Syphilis—Hydrophobia—Glanders 82

CHAPTER VI.

DISEASES OF THE LUNGS AND AIR PASSAGES.

Consumption—Acute Bronchitis-Chronic Bron-
chitis—Asthma—Acute Nasal Catarrh—Ul-
ceration of the Nose—Sore Throat—Quinsy
—Croup—Loss of Voice—Inflammation of
Larynx— Chronic Catarrh — Pneumonia—
Pleurisy 76

CHAPTER VII.

DISEASES OF THE NERVOUS SYSTEM.

Headache—Vertigo—Spinal Irritation—Convulsions—Epilepsy—St. Vitus Dance—Hysteria
Hiccough—Sea Sickness — Neuralgia—Pa-
ralysis. 106

CHAPTER VIII.

DISEASES OF THE HEART.

Palpitation of the Heart—Rheumatism of the Heart—Diseases of the Valves—Enlargement of the Heart—Fatty Degeneration – Angina Pectoris 123

CHAPTER IX.

URINARY DISEASES.

Congestion and Inflammation of the Kidneys— Bright's Disease — Gravel — Retention of Urine—Inflammation of the Bladder—Stone in the Bladder—Involuntary Escape of Urine............................... 130

CHAPTER X.

SPECIAL DISEASES OF MEN.

Gonorrhea, or Clap—Gleet—Balanitis—Phymosis—Paraphimosis—Stricture—Swelled Testicles— Hydrocele —Varicocele— Self-abuse —Spermatorrhea 141

CHAPTER XI.

DISEASES AND INJURIES OF THE SKIN.

Acne, or Flesh Worms—Bed Sores—Boils—Carbuncles — Corns — Chilblains — Dandruff— Falling Out of Hair—Eczema—Freckles— Nettle Rash, or Hives—Prickley Heat— Ring Worm—Salt Rheum—Warts—Itch— Barbers Itch—Burns and Scalds 151

CHAPTER XII.

DISEASES OF WOMEN.

Inflammation of the Vagina—Inflammation and Ulceration of the Womb—Leucorrhea—Displacements of the Womb—Tumors—Cancers—Change of Life.................164

CHAPTER XIII.

THE EYE AND ITS DISORDERS.

The Care of the Eyes—Defects of Vision—The Use of Spectacles—Diseases of the Lids—Weeping, or Watery, Eyes—Cross-Eye—Conjunctivitis—Granular Lids—Ulceration of the Cornea—Opacity of the Cornea—Iritis—Cataract—Glaucoma—Amaurosis .. 178

CHAPTER XIV.

THE EAR AND ITS DISORDERS.

Care of the Ears—Malformations and Injuries of the Ears—Accumulation of Wax—Abscess—Deafness—Polypus.................190

CHAPTER XV.

SURGICAL DISEASES AND ACCIDENTS.

Piles—Fistula of the Anus—Fissure of the Anus—Hernia, or Rupture—Varicose Veins—Ingrown Toe Nails—Diseases of the Bones—Fractures—Sprains—Dislocations- Diseases of the Joints—Spinal Deformities—Knock Knee—Bowed Legs—Club Foot...........196

CHAPTER XVI.

FOOD IN HEALTH AND DISEASE.

Infant Feeding—Food for Adult Life—Food in Old Age—Fallacies Regarding Eating—Diet in Dyspepsia—Food in Biliousness—Food in Nervous Prostration — Food in Rheumatism—Food in Diabetes—Food in Consumption—Diet in Acute Diseases—Food in Convalescence... 212

CHAPTER XVII.

ANTIDOTES FOR POISON.

For Opium—Strychnine—Arsenic—Lead—Aconite—Belladonna—Carbolic Acid—Chloroform—Coal Gas—Illuminating Gas—Oxalic Acid — Gelsemium — Chloral — Poisonous Mushrooms 229

CHAPTER XVIII.

WHAT TO DO IN EMERGENCIES.

For Burns and Scalds—Pistol Wounds—Cuts—Bleeding from the Nose—Bleeding from the Lungs—Fainting—Convulsions—Drowning—Accidents from Collisions 237

CHAPTER I.

The Organs of Digestion.

How to Preserve Health — Diseases of the Digestive Organs — Acute Indigestion — Chronic Dyspepsia—Catarrh of the Stomach—Jaundice — Diarrhea — Chronic Diarrhea—Cholera Morbus—Dysentery—Cholera Infantum — Habitual Constipation — Intestinal Worms.

The organs of the body that take part in preparing and distributing the material necessary to nourish the system are called the organs of digestion. These organs, when spoken of collectively, are called the *digestive* apparatus, which begins with the mouth and ends at the anus, and includes two large collateral structures. Naming them in order we have the mouth, œsophagus or gullet, stomach, small intestines, liver, pancreas or sweet bread, and large intestines.

The mouth first receives the food. Here it is or should be thoroughly masticated, before it is swallowed. This not only prepares it for ready digestion in the stomach, but first mixes it with the saliva, a secretion from several small glands that connect with the mouth by small tubes. The saliva causes a slight change in the food by converting starch into sugar, which is the first change the food undergoes. It also renders swallowing easy. When the food reaches the stomach it stimulates the glands and muscles of that organ, so that the food is moved around, and thoroughly mixed with the gastric juice, which is the digestive fluid of the stomach, and is composed of water, pepsin, lactic acid, and albuminous and salty materials. When acting normally, the articles of food containing albumin—and hence called albuminous substances, such as meats, eggs, milk, and portions of many vegetables—are converted by the gastric juice into a substance called *albuminose*. This, with the starches, sugars, and fats, is now called *chyme*, and passes out of the stomach into the small intestines. The intestines secrete what is called intestinal juice, which, acting on the starch of the chyme, changes it into sugar.

The pancreas produces a secretion of its own, which is emptied through a little canal into the intestines. This secretion is called pancreatic juice, and it acts on the fatty portion of the food, changing it into a substance called chyle.

The liver also empties its secretion—bile—into the intestines, which helps to keep up the motion of the intestines, and also prevents fermentation, thus acting as a valuable auxiliary to digestion.

It will thus be seen that the process of digestion,

which is begun in the stomach, is completed in the intestines. As fast as the digestion is completed, the absorbents of the intestines suck it up, and carry it into the circulation. The fatty portion of the food that has been converted into chyle passes down, and is sucked up by innumerable little vessels called lacteals. These carry it to larger recepticals, and these again to a canal called the *thoracic duct*. This duct conveys material from various parts of the body to be further prepared for use by again passing through the blood. The chyle mixes with this fluid, and is carried into a vein under the left collar bone. From this vein it is carried with the impure blood to the right side of the heart; from that to the lungs, where certain impurities are removed, and thence back to the heart, the motor by which the pure, enriched blood is carried to every part of the body to feed and renew the tissues.

All particles of food that are not acted upon by the digestive fluids pass into the large intestines, and are thrown off from the bowels as effete materials.

It will thus be seen that digestion is a complicated process, and that it must be properly performed in order to keep the entire body in a healthy condition. If digestion is impaired so that food is not supplied in the right form to the blood, the actions of the lungs and heart go on without supplying the tissues with nourishment, and both these organs must soon become diseased in consequence. In short, nearly all functional and many organic diseases owe their beginning to imperfect digestion. How important is it, then, that every one should be familiar with the normal process of digestion, that they might recognize the first symptoms of a departure therefrom.

HOW TO PRESERVE HEALTH.

Those who desire to keep well should be regular in all their habits; should eat a fair quantity of food composed of animal and vegetable products; should never eat so much as to feel uncomfortably full; should chew their food thoroughly before swallowing it; and should take as little fluid as possible till the food is thoroughly masticated and swallowed.

A rest of half an hour after severe physical or mental labor should always be taken before eating, and an hour's rest after a meal is always desirable. If this is not possible, a very light meal should be taken at noon, and the principal meal reserved for the evening, after the work of the day is over. Farmers and all persons engaged in severe physical labor should rest from half an hour to an hour after a midday dinner, which is usually best for them if they can rest before resuming work.

Those suffering from any great mental strain from any cause should abstain from hearty eating, for digestion cannot go on properly during such excitement, and loading the stomach is sure to cause indigestion.

It is better to eat something before retiring than to go to bed hungry. It is also wise for every one to avoid such articles of food as have been found by experience to disagree with them, no matter how wholesome they may be claimed to be.

Many persons, especially those doing mental work, feel the need of some little stimulant. A little light table wine with the meal will be found a valuable aid to such persons, and can be taken with the certainty of deriving benefit from its use.

One of the most important factors in perfect digestion is regular bowels. Every one should so habituate himself that the custom of having the bowels move at a regular hour in the morning becomes a fixed habit. No engagements, however pressing, should interfere with this important call of nature, for when neglected one day, the desire is less the following day, and thus in a short time constipation is established. This is one of the most common causes of deranged digestion. Persons of sedentary habits should take some form of systematic exercise in the open air. Walking is well enough as far as it goes, but it is not enough. The muscles of the arms, chest, and abdomen, should be daily brought into action. Cycling is a most healthful form of exercise for both sexes.*

Bathing is also essential. A free action of the skin relieves the lungs and kidneys of unnecessary work, and prevents the accumulation in the system of effete material. When they can be had, one or two Turkish baths a week will be found specially conducive to health.

Attention to these few suggestions will enable the large majority of people to keep well, for a **per- fect** stomach and liver can always defy disease and the doctors.

The several organs of digestion are liable to be affected by disease, acute or chronic, but as many of them are intricate, and require to be specially examined by the experienced physician, only such as can be easily recognized and treated at home will be considered in these pages. Among those most commonly met with we find acute indigestion, chronic dyspepsia, catarrh of the stomach, torpid liver or biliousness, jaundice, diarrhea, cholera morbus, cholera infantum, dysentery, habitual con- stipation, and intestinal worms all of which we will briefly consider in the order as named.

ACUTE INDIGESTION.

Acute indigestion is usually a temporary dis- turbance of stomach digestion, caused by taking into the stomach some indigestible substance, by over-loading the stomach with too much food, or eating heartily when the system is exhausted by overwork or mental anxiety.

The symptoms are a sharp, cutting pain in the stomach, with a feeling as of a hard lump in the stomach that will not move; sharp spasms of pain, followed by intervals of relaxation; and a bloating or distention of the stomach. These symptoms may show themselves during a meal, immediately after, or an hour or two, after eating.

In severe cases the quickest relief is obtained by swallowing some stimulant. Two tablespoonfuls of good whisky or brandy without water, if possible, is among the best remedies. Ten drops of tincture of red pepper and twenty drops of tincture of ginger in a little water may also be used to advantage by those who object to alcoholic stimulant. This treatment simply stimulates the muscles of the stomach to force the undigested food from the stomach. This will relieve the pain, but the difficulty is not always removed. The natural action of the stomach has been interfered with, and the intestines have more work than their own to perform. Digestion must be promoted and the undigested food must be removed.

As soon as the severe pain is relieved one of the Home Dyspepsia Pills should be taken, and should be continued after each meal for several days. A Home Liver Pill should also be taken at bed time, and repeated every night for several nights if necessary.

CHRONIC DYSPEPSIA.

Chronic dyspepsia is that form of indigestion that has resulted from a depressed or inactive state of the stomach. It is caused by the continued use of improper quality or excessive quantities of food, torpid liver, severe mental or physical effort immediately before or after eating, bad hygienic conditions, or a general depressed state of the system. It is often present in the aged, and may follow as a sequence, after any protracted illness.

Symptoms.—A sense of fullness and weight felt soon after eating, and continuing till the stomach is empty, is the first well defined symptom of this disorder. Following this, wind colic often gives annoyance; there is difficult breathing, palpitation of the heart which is often mistaken for heart disease, constipation, coated tongue, and headache through the temples and eyeballs. The tongue is large and flabby and indented by the teeth around its edges.

When the intestinal digestion is first interfered with the weight and distension are felt below the stomach proper, the lower part of the abdomen is distended with gas, and a constant rumbling is felt in the bowels.

In either case the patient loses strength and flesh, the skin becomes pale and clammy, the hands and feet are cold, despondency ensues, memory is impaired, and all ambition is lost. Of course these are the symptoms of the more serious cases, but every dyspeptic will experience them in time if the disease is not arrested.

Treatment.—The most important thing to consider in the treatment of this disease is the diet. All articles of food containing starch and sugar should, as a rule, be avoided for a time, as these articles, when not digested, readily undergo fermentation, and thus distend the bowels with gas. Among the articles to be avoided are potatoes, corn, rice, white bread, beets, sugar, pastry, puddings, sweetmeats, and the like. Beef and mutton should be well masticated or chopped up fine before cooking, and should always be eaten rare. Milk, eggs, beans, peas, celery, lettuce, tomatoes, graham bread, and bread made from gluten flour may be eaten, but the stomach should never be overloaded. Ripe fruits, in season, are also good as a rule. Any article of food, however, that is known to disagree with a patient should always be avoided, and strong condiments should never be used.

When it does not disagree with a person, a little mild claret wine, taken after a small plate of soup, will be found very beneficial. Aged persons may take about two tablespoonfuls of good whisky or brandy about half an hour before a meal, and be greatly benefited by it.

Next to the diet the condition of the liver and bowels should be considered. If the tongue is coated and the bowels constipated, the Home Liver Pills, used according to directions accompanying them, should be continued till these conditions are corrected. In addition, one Home Dyspepsia Pill should be taken immediately after each meal. In

severe cases, in adults, two pills may often be required at a dose for a week or two.

When there is palpitation of the heart and difficult breathing, speedy relief will often be obtained
by taking twenty drops of essence of peppermint
and as much bicarbonate of soda as can be held on
a ten-cent silver piece. These can be dissolved in
a little water and swallowed.

In all such cases any severe mental strain or
worry will retard recovery, so that in such cases the
above treatment should be followed during a rest
from business cares.

CATARRH OF THE STOMACH.

Catarrh of the stomach, though always causing
indigestion, is different from the dyspepsia just described. It is an inflammation of the membranes
of the stomach, which results, in many cases, in a
thickening of the lining membrane and a congestion
of the bloodvessels of the stomach.

This condition is caused by the continued use of
highly seasoned foods, the excessive use of stimulants, insufficient mastication, overloading the
stomach, the use of very hot or very cold drinks,
and the continued use of morphine or other powerful narcotics.

Sometimes an acute attack may occur, when the
patient will be feverish, the stomach nauseated and
tender on pressure. Great thirst may be present,
and the stomach rejects every thing that enters it.

Such an acute attack may pass into a chronic or long-standing inflammation, but usually the chronic form seems to have been gradually developed from long-continued congestion, without the development of any marked acute symptoms.

Many of the symptoms are the same as those of ordinary dyspepsia. The distention of the stomach and bowels with gases is more marked; and in some cases severe cutting neuralgic pains are produced. Pain is usually present, but at one time it is more severe when the stomach is full, and at another time when it is empty. Acid eructations often rise to the throat, heart-burn and water-brash occur, and in many cases the distress is not relieved till vomiting occurs. In short, all the symptoms of ordinary dyspepsia are present in very aggravated form, with some other distressing ones added.

Treatment.—The same general attention to diet as before described is imperative, and our Home Liver Pills and Home Dyspepsia Pills should be used in ths same way.

In this disease a goblet full of water, as hot as can be swallowed, will be of great value if taken every morning, an hour before breakfast. This warms the stomach, and loosens and removes the thick mucus that has accumulated during the night.

When these cases have been of long standing an experienced physician should be consulted, for it may be necessary to reach the inside of the stomach with medicated injections to prevent the development of ulceration.

TORPID LIVER OR BILIOUSNESS.

By torpid liver is meant a condition in which the bile accumulates in the liver instead of passing into the intestines. This leaves the complexion sallow, causes brown patches to form on the skin, creates a tenderness on pressure along the lower margin of the ribs on the right side, over the liver, and causes pain under or between the shoulderblades. The tongue is coated, the bowels constipated, a feeling of languor and drowsiness is felt, and sleep fails to afford relief from the tired feeling. When these symptoms continue, dyspepsia is sure to follow.

Treatment.—Stimulate the liver to action so that the bile is thrown into the intestines in normal quantity, and the difficulty is removed. This can always be done by the Home Liver Pills, which may confidently be said to be specific for torpid liver. One pill should be taken on going to bed, for several nights in succession. When the bowels move freely more than once a day, a pill should only be taken every second or third night, as required. If one pill at a time does not move the bowels copiously after two or three days, two pills should be taken at a dose, and even three may be taken by some persons. It is always best, however, to commence with one pill, and gradually increase the dose if necessary.

JAUNDICE.

Jaundice is a condition caused by the retention of the bile in a torpid liver to such a degree that it is absorbed into the blood. It imparts the greenish-yellow hue of the bile to the skin, eyes, and other tissues, and hence it is easily recognized.

Treatment.—The free use of the Home Liver Pills should be resorted to at once. A hot lemonade or whisky sling on going to bed—or, what is better, when it can be had, a Turkish bath—will open the pores of the skin and thus help to remove the bile from the blood. A few teaspoonful doses of sweet spirits of nitre to act on the kidneys will also serve a good purpose.

During the continuance of the jaundice it is best to abstain as much as possible from hearty eating.

DIARRHEA.

Simple diarrhea is too well known to require any special description. It is usually met with during the summer season, and indigestible articles of food, with the high temperature. seem to act as exciting causes of the disease. Exposure to cold and damp air, and the sudden arrest of perspiration, also act as exciting causes in producing it.

Bilious diarrhea is a condition to which some people are frequently liable at any season of the year. This is caused when a large quantity of bile passes into the small intestines at once, after its passage had been obstructed for some time.

Treatment.—During an attack of diarrhea it is best to abstain from eating, and also to avoid drinking as much as possible, till the severity of the attack is over. If there is much pain in the bowels, as might be caused by the presence of some undigested portion of food, a dose of castor oil will prove of great service in removing the offending substance. It can be taken with a little coffee, and is not as disagreeable to take as many suppose.

Then the patient should keep as quiet as possible and take one of the Home Cholera Pills every hour till relieved or till five or six doses are taken. After the attack is first controlled, the pills may be continued every three or four hours, if necessary, until there is no likelihood of a recurrence.

Such attacks are apt to leave a person constipated, but this condition is readily overcome by using the Home Liver Pills for a few nights.

CHRONIC DIARRHEA.

Chronic Diarrhea is a name applied to such cases of diarrhea as are of long standing, attacks occurring at short intervals, at all seasons of the year. This is due to deranged conditions of stomach and liver.

None of these cases can be cured by taking the ordinary diarrhea medicines. We must begin right or the disease will continue. Our Dyspepsia Pills should be used after each meal, and the Home Liver Pill at bedtime. If these remedies are followed up for a time the worst cases of chronic diarrhea can be cured.

CHOLERA MORBUS.

Cholera Morbus is an acute inflammation of the lining membrane of the stomach and intestines. It comes on suddenly, and is ushered in by diarrhea, which is soon followed by vomiting. Severe attacks are often mistaken for Asiatic cholera. It may come on at any season of the year, though it is more prevalent in the summer and autumn.

Sudden changes of temperature, prostration from continued heat, the fermentation of undigested foods, drinking ice-water when overheated, and eating unripe fruit or vegetables may give rise to the disorder.

For several days before the attack the patient feels languid and depressed, the tongue is coated, and some diarrhea and slight nausea have been present. Then a chill occurs, usually in the night, and the patient awakes with severe colic and vomiting. The purging then becomes severe, and the patient is greatly prostrated in a short time. Sometimes the attack will come on without warning of any kind. It is severe while it lasts, which may be from a few hours to several days,

Treatment.—To avoid the development of *cholera morbus* all cases of diarrhea should be treated at once with Home Cholera Pills, given according to directions. When the attack has fully developed, small pieces of ice or cold champagne may be given to allay the vomiting, and a mustard poultice, made of equal parts of flour and mustard, should be applied over the stomach and bowels. When the vomiting is allayed the cholera pills should be given, and repeated every half hour for three or four doses, and afterward at longer intervals, as directed in circular. A teaspoonful of good brandy in about the same quantity of water should be given at short intervals till the patient recovers from the extreme prostration.

Where this treatment fails to give prompt relief some other complication is sure to be present, and a physician should be called without delay.

After the attack is over the liver usually becomes torpid and the bowels constipated. In such condition our Home Liver Pill should be used.

DYSENTERY.

Dysentery differs from the diseases above described by being an inflammation and ulceration of the large intestines. It is caused by the same general conditions as develop the diseases of other portions of the bowels, but is influenced by malarial conditions to such an extent as to develop it as an epidemic,

It begins about the same as an ordinary diarrhea, but the discharges soon have a sticky white
appearance, and finally they become bloody. It is
this that has given to the disease the name of
" bloody flux."

The first symptoms closely resemble those of
cholera morbus, without much nausea, but soon
severe colicky pains are felt on either side of the
abdomen above the groin; there is a feeling of
pressure and uneasiness in the lower bowel, and a
spasm at the anus (back passage), which is intensely
painful. The discharges, of a jelly-like mucus, are
streaked with blood at first, but when the disease
continues they appear almost like pure blood, and
are very frequent.

In most cases there will be considerable fever,
which is likely to come on at a certain time of the
day, most usually in the afternoon. It lasts for
several hours and then subsides.

Treatment.—At the onset of the disease our
Cholera Pill should be used freely. Two pills may
be given at a dose, and repeated in half an hour.
After the second dose, they should not be taken
oftener than once in two hours.

If there is much fever twenty drops of tincture
of aconite root should be put in a goblet with six
tablespoonfuls of water, and a teaspoonful given
from the goblet every half hour till the fever subsides.

The diet should be milk, with one-quarter lime-water added, beef juice, raw oysters if fresh, eggs, egg-nog (made with eggs, brandy, and milk), custard, etc. Solid foods should be avoided.

Sometimes it is necessary to make a starch solution of the consistency of syrup, and to add to half a pint a teaspoonful of laudanum, and inject that quantity into the rectum with a Davidson syringe. The patient should rest on the left side, and after using the injection a napkin should be pressed against the anus to prevent the starch solution from escaping at once.

After the bowel trouble subsides, Home Malaria Pills should be taken for a week or ten days, or longer, if the patient does not regain strength speedily.

CHOLERA INFANTUM.

Cholera Infantum is a name applied to an inflammation of the lining membrane of the stomach and intestines of children, which usually occurs during the teething period. It is analogous to cholera morbus in the adult, and is attended by vomiting, purging, and considerable fever. It is often called "summer cholera" and "summer complaint."

The disease occurs in young infants when the mother's milk is defective in quality, or when the child is fed from the bottle with improperly prepared food. It is, however, more common at the age of teething, when the nervous system has been irritated, and when children are allowed to eat considerable bread, potatoes, sweets, and such articles as the system is not yet capable of digesting.

The restlessness, irritability, and feverishness, that precede an attack are so well known to every mother that they need no description here. The bowels may be loose for several days before vomiting sets in, though vomiting and purging will often begin at once without much previous disturbance.

The discharges from the bowels soon become watery, and are greenish or greenish-yellow in color. The abdomen is tender to the touch, the legs are drawn up, and the slightest motion causes pain, and the child to cry out or moan. Nothing will remain on the stomach, and the retching is often severe. The child soon looks thin in the face and body, the eyes are sunken and half closed, the mouth is partly open, and the lips are dry and cracked.

The disease often develops inflammation of the covering of the spinal cord and brain, when the back of the head becomes extremely hot, the head moves incessantly, and the child sinks into a stupor and dies.

This disease is most frequently developed as a result of ignorance of the parents in regard to the proper way to feed children under four years of age. For full directions on this subject see article on " Infant Feeding " in this manual,

Treatment.—Attention to what is taken into the atomach is the first consideration in the treatment of this disease. Nourishment either from the breast or bottle should be given at longer intervals than usual, and should be much less than usual in quantity. Small pieces of ice to suck should be substituted for large draughts of water. See article on " Infant Feeding " for preparation of milk as a substitute for mother's milk. Bathing two or three times a day in water at 100° at first and gradually cooled to 80° materially aids in reducing the fever, and is grateful to the child.

The vomiting is often allayed by from ten to twenty drops of pure brandy, given in water, every two, three, or four, hours.

In the way of medicines the following will be found very serviceable in promptly relieving the disease in the majority of cases: To eight table-spoonfuls of water in a goblet add six drops of tincture of aconite root. To another goblet with the same quantity of water add ten drops of tincture of ipecac and five drops of tincture of nux vomica. Commence by giving a teaspoonful from the first goblet, and fifteen minutes after a teaspoonful from the second goblet. Continue alternating the medicine, one being given after the other with fifteen minutes between doses. When the fever subsides the doses can be given half an hour apart, and as the symptoms improve longer intervals should pass between doses. The child should not be disturbed when asleep. This treatment, with attention to diet, will cure even severe cases.

When the head symptoms are present, ten drops of tincture of gelsemium should be substituted for the tincture of aconite, and the doses alternated as before.

In all severe cases it is best to send for a physician.

HABITUAL CONSTIPATION.

As constipation is always associated with some other derangement, it is important always to ascertain and remove the cause, if possible. Attention to diet is of the first importance, and on this point the reader is referred to the directions regarding the same as given in Chapter XVI.

Our Home Liver Pills, when taken according to directions, will overcome the worst cases of habitual constipation. Rowing, a gentle lifting exercise, or any motion, that will bring all the muscles of the body into action, will be found a great help in the right direction. Gently kneading and rubbing over the surface of the bowels, for twenty minutes every morning, will also materially help. Regularity as to the time of going to stool must not be forgotten either, for a neglect of this necessary precaution will greatly retard the desired regularity in the action of the bowels.

By following these directions and taking the

pills till the bowels move freely and the tongue is no longer coated the constipation can be cured. For a few days after discontinuing the pills, there may be a slight tendency to constipation, but if the effort to secure a motion is followed every day, the bowels will become as regular as clock-work.

INTESTINAL WORMS.

Worms of various kinds are produced and developed in the human body, and this remarkable fact constitutes one of the most interesting and astonishing studies in connection with medical science. They are found in many of the organs and tissues of the body, but are most frequently met with in the digestive canal.

It may be interesting to know that thirty different kinds of worms are known to infest the human body under varying conditions. Of these, three kinds are often met with in the intestines, and are known as round or stomach worms, thread-worms and tape-worms. It is with these only that we will deal at present.

The presence of worms in the bowels is made manifest by the following symptoms: paleness of the face which sometimes changes to a dirty red or bluish hue, dark circles around the eyes, itching of the nostrils and anus (back passage), disturbed sleep, grinding of the teeth during sleep, swelling of the abdomen, griping pains in the bowels, and slimy stools, which are very irregular. The appetite varies greatly, being voracious at one time and ca-pricious at another.

Though these symptoms point to the presence of worms, they are not always reliable. The only cer-tainty is the presence of worms or parts of them in the passages from the bowels.

Round-worms vary in length from six to ten inches, and in general appearance closely resemble the earth worm commonly used as a bait while fish-ing. They are present in the small intestines of children and sickly persons who are badly fed.

The swollen abdomen, colicky pains, slimy pas-sages from the bowels, and the peculiarly disagree-able breath at once suggest the presence of round worms.

The *thread-worms*, or pin worms, as the smaller ones are called, are usually found in the lower bowel, and may often be seen on the surface of the skin, having worked themselves through the anus. They will even extend and find their way into the vagina in female children, and produce a whitish discharge, the cause of which often remains a mys-tery. They will sometimes form in solid bunches, which materially interfere with the natural action of the bowels.

These worms cause a feeling of fullness and pressure in the rectum, extreme itching at and around the fundament, oozing of slimy matter, irri-table temper, and at times great depression of spirits.

Tape-worm is found in the small intestines, and varies from a few feet to twenty or thirty yards in length. It is flat, and formed of numerous pieces ranging from one-eighth to one-half inch in length, and nearly as broad, which are joined together by joints resembling those of sugar cane. The tape-worm is more commonly met with in adults, while the other two varieties are incidental to childhood. The latter occur in great numbers while the tape-worm is usually single. The general symptoms already given are usually present, and in addition the sufferer eats voraciously, is always hungry, but remains thin and lean. There is no certain symptom, however, of the presence of the tape-worm except when sections of it are passed from the bowels.

Treatment.—In treating round-worms and thread-worms the patient should abstain from eating during the greater portion of the day and before going to bed. Home Worm Lozenges should be given, according to directions. The following morning from one teaspoonful to a tablespoonful of castor oil, with from ten to thirty drops of oil of turpentine should be administered before breakfast, the dose being regulated according to the age. There is no better remedy for this purpose than this old-fashioned, much-despised castor oil. If worms are present they are pretty certain to be passed with the first motion of the bowels. If no worms appear, the treatment may be tried again in a few days.

The thread-worms are often best removed by an

injection into the rectum of a strong solution of warm salt and water, in addition to the above treatment.

In the treatment of tape-worm a great variety of remedies have been recommended, but the most effectual is the oil of male-fern. After fasting for twelve hours, a tablespoonful of oil of male-fern, mixed with two tablespoonfuls of syrup, should be taken at bed-time. The following morning an ounce of castor oil, with a teaspoonful of the oil of turpentine, should be taken before breakfast. If there is any tape-worm present this treatment will certainly remove it, but a second trial may be necessary before the entire worm is expelled. The worm should be examined to ascertain if the head is expelled, for if it is not it will be rapidly reproduced.

CHAPTER II.

Malarial Diseases.

MALARIAL FEVERS—INTERMITTENT FEVER—REMIT-
TENT, OR BILIOUS, FEVER.

Under the general heading of Malarial Diseases
are included all those disorders that are known to
be produced by the absorption into the system of a
poisonous germ from the atmosphere which is commonly called malaria, or marsh-miasm. It has
been demonstrated that in certain seasons of the
year, and in some regions of country where vegetable substances have been under moisture for a
time, and then exposed to the rays of the sun,
minute disease germs are produced in such quantities as to poison the atmosphere for a considerable
distance around. This condition occurs in low-
lying swampy ground, where fresh water abounds,
and is more common in the summer and fall.
Digging up and exposing fresh earth to any extent
also develops or liberates these germs.

While there can be no mistaking the symptoms
of true malaria, it is nevertheless true that the
term malaria is often so loosely used as to be ap-

plied to any condition for which the doctor cannot find a better term.

The absorption of the malaria germs by the system produces conditions which vary in proportion to the amount of absorption which has taken place. The symptoms may vary from slight languor and chilliness, to the most violent ague and fever, and different names have been applied to the different conditions developed, As a rule, a healthy, robust person may be exposed to a malarious atmosphere for a long time without being affected in the least thereby; while a person in poor health or with a torpid liver is very likely to suffer from some malarial disease.

MALARIAL FEVERS

Malarial fevers are properly divided into two kinds, viz., intermittent and remittent fevers; but these have received different names by which they are often popularly known.

Intermittent fever is of malarial origin, and receives its name from the fact that it occurs periodically, leaving the patient comparatively well between the attacks. It begins with a chill and cold stage, which is followed by a hot stage, and that again by a sweating stage.

It is variously called chills, fever and ague, but more properly ague and fever, and dumb ague. These names owe their origin to the several symptoms developed by the varying degrees of severity of the disease. When there is a feeling of languor, with frequent recurrences of slight chills, followed by flashes of heat, the term "chills" is applied; when there is a continued cold stage with slight fever following, and little or no sweating, it is called dumb ague; but when there is a pronounced chill, continued from half an hour to an hour or two, with feeling of intense cold, and this is followed by a high fever, which lasts as long, and finally gives way to profuse sweating, we have a fully developed intermittent fever, or ague and fever.

When the sweating stage is over, the patient feels almost as well as usual, but after a certain regular interval the paroxysm recurs and takes the same course as before. Sometimes the attacks come on every day, while they may only recur every second, third, or fourth day. Whatever the interval may be the paroxysms, when renewed, follow the same course as at first. In many cases the disease is so persistent and severe that the patient is entirely worn out and life becomes a burden.

Many times, before this disease is fully developed, the patient suffers from general languor and depression of spirit, has a continuous headache, pains in the muscles, coated tongue, and constipated bowels.

These symptoms, especially in malarial districts, should be sufficient warning, and some preventive treatment should be at once adopted.

Remittent fever, also called bilious fever, and bilious remittent fever, is only another form of malaria. The cause that produces it, the premonitory symptoms, and the ushering in of the attack are about the same as met with in intermittent fever. When the attack is once developed, however, the disease continues till it is broken up by treatment, or runs its course. At a certain hour every day, or every other, there is a remission of the fever, marked by slight perspiration. This lasts for a short time, and the fever again manifests itself as before. In mild cases the remission is of longer duration, and a chill ushers in the next paroxysm. In severe cases, however, the fever is almost continuous, and often assumes a low, typhoid type, which may at any time prove fatal.

Treatment.—All treatment of malarial fevers must have in view the relief of the patient during the paroxysm, the prevention of a recurrence, and destroying the poison in the system, so as to effect a permanent cure.

When the first symptoms are felt, and before the chill or fever occurs, the Home Malaria Pill should be taken. It will also be found necessary to promote a good action on the liver by the use of the Home Liver Pill. Both these remedies should be used continuously till all the symptoms have entirely disappeared. Even then the malaria pill should be taken for three days of each week for four weeks to prevent a relapse. This has been found necessary on account of a tendency to a recurrence of malaria every seventh, fourteenth, twenty-first, and twenty-eighth days. No malarial medicine should be given during the chill or fever.

During the continuance of the cold stage the patient should be well covered up in bed, with hot bottles or irons to the feet and hands, if desired.

When the hot stage comes on all extra bed-clothing should be removed. Cool drinks may be given, and in severe cases the skin may be bathed with water at about eighty degrees temperature.

To shorten the febrile stage and render the patient more comfortable, three drops of the tincture of gelsemium should be given in a teaspoonful of water every fifteen or twenty minutes till perspiration commences. This treatment will materially shorten the hot stage.

For the sweating stage nothing can be done but to wipe the body with a towel, and to give the patient whatever drink may be desired.

Should one malaria pill every three hours fail to prevent a recurrence of a second paroxysm, two pills should be taken every three hours.

CHAPTER III.

Specific Germ Diseases.

SMALL-POX—CHICKEN-POX— MEASLES—ERYSIPELAS
—CHOLERA—YELLOW FEVER—DIPHTHERIA-LA
GRIPPE, OR INFLUENZA—HAY FEVER—WHOOP-
ING COUGH—MUMPS—TYPHOID FEVER.

Modern science has demonstrated that a large
number of our most fatal, as well as most prevalent
diseases, are due to the inhaling and absorbing of
certain specific germs from the atmosphere. Some
go so far as to say that all diseases are caused by
disease germs, but this claim cannot be verified by
any satisfactory proof. There are, however, enough
of such diseases about which there is no dispute,
and these we will briefly describe without any attempt at special qualification.

Small-pox, chicken-pox, measles, German measles, scarlet fever, and erysipelas, are usually described as eruptive fevers; while cholera, diphtheria, influenza, hay fever, whooping cough, and
mumps, are classed as miasmatic diseases.

Whatever may be the character of the specific
poisons or germs that produce these diseases, cer-

tain it is that nature makes an effort to rid the system from the intruders, and thus the symptoms of
the various diseases are produced. It is therefore
necessary to direct all efforts in the line of treatment to the destruction of the specific germs.

SMALL-POX.

Small-pox is an eruptive disease, especially contagious in character.

The first symptoms are languor and depression,
such as precedes all fevers, intense pain in the
back and legs, with severe headache. After a few
days a severe chill is felt, and then a high fever
sets in, and lasts for three or four days. An eruption shows itself at this time, when the fever and
pain in the back and head are all relieved. The
eruption at first consists of slightly elevated red
points, which are somewhat hard, and feel like
small shot under the finger. The second day after
the eruption appears the red points enlarge, and
look like inflamed pimples, and by the third day a
clear fluid is seen under a delicate vesicle. In
about two days more the top of each vesicle has
the appearance of a pimple filled with pus, or matter; when full, the vesicle flattens and falls in till a
marked depression is formed.

It is only after the vesicle forms that the disease
can be communicated, and usually from eight to
fourteen days may intervene after exposure before
the first symptoms begin to show themselves.

Some claim that persons who have been vaccinated have a milder form of the disease, which is called varioloid. This is a fallacy, and we believe the day is not far distant when vaccination will be abandoned in all civilized countries.

Treatment.—It has long been known that oxygen destroys minute germs of all kinds, and the aim has always been to supply extra oxygen to the blood in some way. Little success had been attained however, until concentrated oxygen in the form of ozone was manufactured, so that water could be strongly charged with it. This has been successfully done in Germany, and the process with the complete apparatus was obtained at great expense and brought to America, and the Home Treatment has now the exclusive right to manufacture ozone water by the only method by which ozone can be utilized in the treatment of disease.

In ozone, therefore, we have a specific in the treatment of small-pox and all other diseases that are caused by disease germs. It should be taken internally, as well as used to wash the pustules. If the pustules are not rubbed or scratched, and the ozone water is applied freely several times a day, the patient is made very comfortable, and pitting is prevented.

During the prevalence of small-pox ozone vapor should be generated in the rooms, and if a person has been exposed the water should be drank freely, according to directions.

For full particulars of this wonderful agent, carefully read the article on ozone in this Manual.

CHICKEN-POX.

Chicken-pox is a very mild form of eruptive fever which is generally met with in childhood. An eruption on the body is the first symptom to attract attention. Its appearance is that of a crop of small water blisters, which soon extend to the extremities. There is a slight fever manifest about the same time as the appearance of the eruption. The vesicles dry up and fall off in from three to five days, and the fever then disappears.

There is no special treatment necessary, except to avoid exposure to cold during the continuance of the eruption.

MEASLES.

Measles is well known to almost every mother. It is easily communicated from one person to another, and is believed by many to be in the atmosphere. It certainly occurs epidemically, and will often attack children who have not been directly exposed.

The period of incubation ranges from twelve to fourteen days. The disease is one especially of childhood, though adults are also frequently attacked by it, and one attack does not necessarily prevent another.

A feeling of languor, muscular soreness, headache and backache, followed by frequent chills, or on the third or fourth day by a pronounced rigor and fever, are the first symptoms. The eyes, nose, and throat, are also inflamed, and the eyes and nose usually discharge a watery secretion. The first symptoms are often so severe that the nature of the disease cannot be determined till the eruption appears.

On the fourth day the eruption appears, and as it develops the fever subsides. The eruption is elevated under the skin, and the elevated spots are red, but begin to fade about the seventh day.

Treatment.—Little can be done to relieve the patient during the initial stage except to keep him quiet in bed. After the fever develops warm drinks should be used freely to promote the eruption, and the body can be frequently bathed with equal parts of hot water and ozone water. The ozone water should be taken internally as soon as the first symptoms appear. Where there are other children they should take the ozone water as a preventive, and the rooms should be thoroughly disinfected with ozone vapor.

For full particulars carefully read article on ozone in this Manual.

SCARLET FEVER.

Scarlet fever is another of the contagious diseases that is developed by a specific germ poison,

It is the most serious, and proves the most fatal of all the diseases of its class.

The premonitory symptoms are about the same as those met with in the other eruptive fevers. In most cases there is a marked inflammation with soreness of the throat.

The fever is generally continuous and severe, and the eruption, which appears at the end of the first or beginning of the second day, is a pale red at first but soon becomes almost scarlet, and spreads rapidly over the entire body. The eruption fades away after from three to seven days, and the entire outer skin peals off in scales.

Treatment.—This disease should always be attended by a physician. The free use of ozone water from the beginning and the generating of ozone in the sick room should be kept up, no matter what other treatment may be employed. Warm drinks and milk punch are of great service in promoting the eruption and keeping up the strength. A teaspoonful of powdered borax and the same amount of salt, dissolved in a gobletful of ozone water, should be used freely as a gargle, when the throat is inflamed.

After the disease is over, if there is a discharge from the ear or an inflammation of the eyes, an experienced surgeon should be consulted without delay, as neglect of these common sequences often results in loss of sight or hearing.

See article on ozone in this Manual.

ERYSIPELAS.

Erysipelas is now recognized as a disease of the blood, produced by a specific germ, though many have considered it especially a disease of the skin.

It begins with the same symptoms as the other eruptive fevers, and after the fever begins an inflamed point is seen on the face or some other part of the body. It spreads rapidly, presents a livid red appearance, with a thickening and hardness of the affected part. The pain is of a burning, scalding character, and the fever is often very severe.

Treatment.—Here, too, the internal use of ozone water is valuable, and the best external application that can be used is sheets of absorbent cotton or carded wool saturated in the ozone water. It is always best after the first application to moisten the cotton without removing it, thus more effectually excluding the air from the inflamed surface.

Dialysed iron should be given in half teaspoonful doses, in water, four or five times a day, and in some cases our malaria pill will prove of great benefit while the patient is recovering from his attack.

CHOLERA.

Cholera is an epidemic infectious disease, which is characterized by vomiting and purging, and a final condition of collapse, which usually results in death. In some cases a reaction occurs after the relapse and the patient slowly improves and finally recovers. It is spoken of as Asiatic cholera, and epidemic cholera. It is generally admitted at the present day that this disease is propagated by a minute organism which is popularly called a cholera germ. Fortunately the disease seldom reaches this country, and when it does, with our improved quarantine and hygienic regulations, its spread is limited to a comparatively small territory.

Most cases of cholera begin with ordinary diarrhea, which if permitted to continue, will develop into a genuine case of cholera. When the disease is prevalent this diarrhea, at first simple, soon assumes the type of cholera morbus, and after a few days there is a marked degree of chilliness and a sense of anxiety or fear seizes the patient. The discharges from the bowels and stomach come on with great force and are very copious. They have a grayish-whitish appearance and are often spoken of as rice-water discharges. There is intense thirst, the tongue is cold and has a white pasty coating, the countenance is sunken and of a leaden hue, the nose is pinched, the eyes staring, and the breath cool. Cramps are soon felt in the legs, arms, and the muscles of the back and abdomen; the skin becomes cold and covered with a sticky perspiration; the fingers, nose, and lips, assume a blue color, rings form around the eyes, the urine is suppressed or greatly diminished, and complete collapse occurs, and death takes place in from twenty to forty-eight hours from the first onset of the disease. In some instances, death may occur in two or three hours.

Treatment.—During the prevalence of cholera, no case of diarrhea, however slight, should be overlooked, and the greatest precaution should be taken regarding diet. Unripe fruit and vegetables should be carefully avoided, moderate quantities only of the most nutritious foods should be taken, irregular habits, excessive use of stimulants, and exhaustion from over-work, should be carefully avoided. The discharges from cholera patients should be immediately removed and thoroughly disinfected with strong carbolic acid or some agent equally as powerful. Not only the houses in which cholera existed, but all houses in the neighborhood, should be thoroughly fumigated with ozone vapor, and ozone water should be freely drank in preference to that from the ordinary water supply. By these means the cholera germs are destroyed and thus prevented from impregnating the atmosphere, and the use of the ozone water will prevent their introduction into the system.

At the first appearance of the diarrhea Home Cholera Pills should be used freely, according to directions, the patient should be kept quiet, mustard should be applied over the stomach and abdomen, and the fears of the patient should be allayed as much as possible. When evidence of collapse begins, brandy should be freely administered by the mouth, or if it cannot be retained, it should be injected under the skin. It should be, however, borne in mind that in all cases of cholera the family physician should be called at the early stage of the disease.

DIPHTHERIA.

Diphtheria is an acute, contagious disease, caused by specific disease germs, which poison the system and develop local manifestations in the throat, with enlargement of the tonsils and other glands of the neck. The throat affection is in the form of an ulceration, which is soon covered by a whitish or brownish exudation.

.The first symptoms of the disease are those of languor and depression, which may last for several days. In some cases there are the ordinary symptoms of catarrh present, with heat, irritation, and pain in the throat, with much soreness on attempting to swallow. In two or three days a chilly feeling is developed, or a pronounced rigor may occur; this is followed by fever, headache, backache, and muscular pains. In some cases these symptoms are very violent, and in others comparatively mild. The tongue is covered with a thick white coating, and the tonsils and back part of the throat are covered with grayish white patches. These rapidly extend over the entire throat, and form a false membrane which would soon obstruct the air passages. In many cases the patient will not complain of sore throat until the disease is well developed, and extensive ulceration will be found in the throat on the first examination. The exudation in the throat itself forms a poison, and if not removed, absorption into the blood takes place from it, and more serious symptoms are developed.

Treatment.—Ozone water will be found of great advantage both in the treatment of this disease and as a prevention against it when it prevails in any locality. It should be drank freely, and can be used as a gargle or with a spraying apparatus for the throat every hour or two during the day. When the ulceration first appears, its spread can be arrested and its virulence destroyed by the application of carbolic acid with a camel's-hair brush. Two teaspoonfuls of pure carbolic acid should be added to one teaspoonful of glycerine. With the tongue well depressed with a spoon, this mixture should be freely applied to the ulcerated parts, care being taken not to have enough on the brush to allow it to run down the throat and burn unaffected parts.

In cases where the fever is high, benefit will be derived from the use of the following: Tincture of veratrum viride (Norwoods'), three drops; water, six ounces, or twelve tablespoonfuls. Of this a teaspoonful can be given to children over three years of age, at intervals of half an hour's time, till the skin becomes moist, and slight nausea is produced. Adults should take two teaspoonfuls in the same manner. As the disease passes off the patient is greatly prostrated, and therefore milk punch, beef juice, and the most nutritious and easily digested food, should be given, both during and after the disease. As a general tonic our Malaria Pill will serve a good purpose until the patient has fully recovered strength.

LA GRIPPE—INFLUENZA.

La Grippe is the French name given to epidemic Influenza. It is due to the presence in the atmosphere of a specific germ, and is analogous to similar diseases which often prevail among horses, and is called an *epizootic*, which simply means " upon the horse," as epidemic means " upon the people."

The disease begins suddenly with a decided chill, or chilliness, alternating with flashes of heat. The fever follows the chill at once, and in some cases is very severe. There is usually severe pain in the back, and muscular pains in the arms and legs, with headache in the front part of the head and through the eyes. The nose, throat, and eyes, are usually hot and red, the voice is husky, and a dry, troublesome cough is present. After a few days a free, thin, and acrid discharge escapes from the nose and throat, and a purulent matter is thrown off with each fit of coughing. In some cases incessant sneezing is a common symptom at first, but this disappears after the discharge begins. Extreme prostration always follows an attack of *la grippe*, and pneumonia is liable to set in on the slightest exposure to cold.

Treatment.—At the outset of the disease a hot

lemonade, with an ounce of good whiskey or brandy, will often produce a favorable effect. A generous diet and moderate use of milk punch will be found of great benefit through the entire disease. To control the fever twenty drops of tincture of aconite root should be put in a goblet of water, and of this a teaspoonful should be taken every hour until the fever subsides. To relieve the inflammation of the nose and throat, our improved Home Inhaler, with inhalation No. 2 accompanying it, should be used for two or three minutes at a time, once every two or three hours. For violent headache, which is so prominent in severe cases and severe muscular pains our Neurodine Tablet is especially serviceable. When taken according to directions, it will not only relieve the pain but also the congestion and irritation of the nerve centers, upon which so much of the distress of this disease depends. In all cases of la grippe it is important that the atmosphere of the room should be moist. For this purpose arrangements should be made by which steam escaping from boiling water should be provided.

HAY FEVER.

Hay fever is a distressing acute, catarrhal condition affecting the mucous membrane of the nose and throat. It is due to a specific disease germ, usually developed during summer and fall. Some persons are particularly liable to be attacked by it at or about the same time every year. Among the other names by which it is known are hay asthma, rose cold, June cold, and autumnal catarrh. Like all specific diseases, an attack of hay fever is preceded by a feeling of lassitude and weariness, loss of appetite and coated tongue, although in some cases it comes on suddenly. Those who are subject to it have no difficulty in recognizing the earliest symptoms. These are an itching or burning sensation in the eyes, nose, and back part of the throat, which is soon followed by the discharge of a clear, watery fluid, and by frequent and violent sneezing. So severe is the inflammation at times that the eyes become red and swollen, and the passages to the nose are almost entirely obstructed. The throat is hot, dry, and swollen, and the passages to the ears are also involved so as frequently to obstruct the hearing. In the severer forms of the disease the inflammation extends downward to the air passages of the lungs, thus occasioning extreme difficulty of breathing, resembling asthma, which is accompanied by a wheezy or croupy cough. In these cases the patient cannot lie down, feels as if he cannot breathe, becomes pale and exhausted, and covered with cold perspiration. These sometimes will be relieved for a short period, but will begin again with increased severity. As a rule the general system does not suffer materially, except when the patient loses rest from the severity of the local symptoms.

Treatment.—For most people who are liable to

attacks of hay fever a change of climate is always of great advantage, although it is not always easy to know what change is the best. One person is entirely relieved by a sojourn to the White Mountains, the Catskills, or Adirondacks, while others find a sea voyage the most beneficial.

In the way of medicines both internal and external, about every variety has been used, but few have seemed to reach the difficulty so as to allay the distressing symptoms. A remedy that will permanently relieve one person may have little or no effect upon another; so that the aim should always be to employ such remedies as will have a tendency to destroy this specific hay fever germ, both locally and constitutionally. Again we have to recommend ozone water to be drank freely, so that the concentrated ozone thus introduced into the system will have the effect of destroying the minute organisms that give rise to the disease. After many years of careful observation, we have found that our Inhalent No. 2, used in our improved Home Inhaler, has the best and speediest effect in relieving the disease of anything we can try. This inhalation should be used as soon as the first symptoms manifest themselves, and should be regularly continued at short intervals until the inflammatory symptoms have entirely disappeared. We have known many cases to be cut short and their occurrence prevented by this treatment, and in all cases the symptoms are greatly modified.

WHOOPING-COUGH.

Whooping-cough is a disease of childhood, characterized by forcible spasmodic expiration, and a
peculiar whoop or cough, attending the inhalation
of air into the lungs.

Its general symptoms are two well known to require special mention. The disease is contagious,
and only occurs, as a rule, once in a lifetime. At
first the symptoms are those of an ordinary cold in
the head with a slight cold in the throat and a
feeling of general languor and loss of appetite.
After a week or two paroxysms of the peculiar
cough, which consists of short expulsions of air,
take place. While coughing the face gets red,
the eyes swollen and bulging, the body bent
forward, and with each paroxysm the breath is
almost exhausted. When the disease occurs in the
summer or early fall, it is mild and lasts but a short
time, but if it extends into the cold weather the at
tack is greatly prolonged, and the cough may continue the entire winter.

Treatment.—This is another of the diseases in
which medicines have not been very satisfactorily
used. Change of air is usually beneficial, but this
can seldom be secured. Quiet should be obtained
at night, if possible, and for this purpose the following mixture will be found beneficial: Tincture
of gelsemium, ten drops; tincture of aconite root,
six drops; tincture of lobelia, twenty drops; water ·

eight tablespoonfuls. Of this a teaspoonful may be given every hour to a child between one and three years of age, while those over three years can take two teaspoonfuls at same intervals. After six or eight doses have been given in succession, it should be discontinued for several hours. The sleeping rooms should be thoroughly impregnated with ozone vapor in order to thoroughly destroy the atmospheric germs. Attention must also be given to frequent bathing, with the precaution that the child is not afterward exposed to cold. In cases of long standing the following mixture should be used: iodide of potash, one drachm; syrup, two tablespoonfuls; water, six tablespoonfuls; of which give a teaspoonful every three or four hours. This remedy will reduce the chronic thickening of the membranes and prevent the accumulating of the tenacious mucus, which so frequently causes the child to vomit before it is freed from the throat by the paroxysms of coughing.

MUMPS.

Mumps is a specific inflammation of the large glands under the ear, known as the parotid glands. It also belongs to the class of diseases caused by specific air germs. It usually occurs as an epidemic, and is ushered in by a feeling of languor and weariness, followed, after two or three days, by a chill and slight fever. It is more frequently met with in males than in females, and usually at-

tacks those from five to fifteen years of age. · From
twelve to twenty-four hours after the chill a sharp
pain is felt behind the jaw and under the ear, which
extends into the throat and to the ear. A prominent swelling is soon recognized so as to form a
marked protuberance in front of and below the ear.
It is very sensitive to the touch; the jaw becomes
stiff, and sometimes the swelling and pain extends
to the glands under the arm and even to the arm
itself. It reaches its hight in from three to five
days, then remains stationary for a day or two, and
then rapidly diminishes, so that it has entirely disappeared from the neck by the twelfth day. Sometimes only one side is affected, while again the inflammation will occur on both sides simultaneously,
or will begin on one side and only attack the other
when the swelling of the first begins to disappear.
The swelling will sometimes suddenly leave the
glands of the neck and attack the glands of some
remote part of the body, as the breasts or testicles.
The inflammation in the new seat of the disease
will be severe for a time, when it will suddenly disappear from there, and again show itself in the neck.

Treatment.—The patient should be kept within
doors and free from all exposure to cold or
draughts. To remove the pain, warm applications
applied to the seat of the swelling is best. When
the pain is unbearable one of our Neurodine Tablets
may be given at bedtime and repeated in a couple
of hours, if necessary, to quiet the patient. A

Seidlitz's Powder given in the morning to relieve the bowels, and occasionally a sponge bath with tepid water will also be found beneficial. A hot lemonade on going to bed will promote perspiration, and in that way give relief. No other treatment is necessary as the disease is of short duration and is rarely attended by any serious complications.

TYPHOID FEVER.

Typhoid fever is a name given to an acute febrile disease which is characterized by an inflammation and ulceration of some of the glands of the intestines, and in most instances has a peculiar eruption on the abdomen. It is generally considered to be due to some peculiar poison, the exact nature of which has not yet been ascertained. The poison is supposed to emanate from animal decomposition, but certain conditions are necessary to produce the typhoid germ. It should always be borne in mind that the discharges from typhoid patients should not be thrown into cesspools, but should be thoroughly disinfected and removed to some distance. The disease is unquestionably contagious in a feeble degree, but is most liable to be produced by the development of germs from the continued fermentation of the discharges of the patient than from contact with the person. Sometimes an ordinary case of malarial fever will run along for a few weeks and then develop into the peculiar symptoms of typhoid fever.

For a week or ten days prior to the setting in of the disease the patient feels depressed, and tires easily over the slightest exertion. Headache, poor appetite, a slight diarrhea, and even bleeding from the nose, are sometimes noticed. The patient with difficulty applies himself to any mental work, and sleep is disturbed and unrefreshing. Then for several days a feeling of chilliness will occur at different times, and finally the fever begins. In some cases the disease sets in with a disgust for food, extreme nausea, and even vomiting and diarrhea. The fever usually runs high, the patient is generally prostrated both physically and mentally, and this condition continues through the disease, which is apt to run its course in about three weeks. From the seventh to the tenth day there is marked disturbance of mind which is characterized by delirium, picking at the bedclothes and at imaginary objects in the air, and trembling of the muscles. An eruption of isolated spots, about as big as a pinhead, begins to show itself over the abdomen about the same time. This eruption may be very profuse, sparsely scattered over the body, or entirely absent. The abdomen is distended enormously with gases, yields a hollow sound when tapped with the finger, and is usually extremely hot. This is due to the fact that the principal seat of the disease is in the lining membrane of the bowels, and when cases terminate fatally it is from a perforation of the bowels at the seat of the disease,

Treatment. — It is important to keep up the strength of the patient in typhoid fever. With this object in view, milk and lime water, milk punches, beef juice, and alcoholic stimulants have to be resorted to and continued throughout the disease. The fever is best controlled by the following: Tincture of gelsemium, one drachm; tincture of veratrum veride, thirty drops; water, eight tablespoonfuls. Mix in a goblet and give one teaspoonful every hour until the skin becomes slightly moist or the patient feels more comfortable. Frequent sponge baths are essential to keep the skin active, and are very grateful to the patient. A tablespoonful of sweet olive oil with ten drops of oil of turpentine may be given three times a day with advantage. Warm fermentation of hops should be continually applied over the abdomen for the purpose of allaying the local inflammation and preventing the ulceration of the bowels. During the continuance of the disease our Malaria Pill should be given at least three times a day, and after the fever is broken up nothing will so speedily restore the patient's prostrated nervous system as our Nerve Tonic Pills. This last mentioned pill, with the most nutritious diet, milk, eggs, and brandy, should be judiciously and frequently administered, during convalescence, so as to build up the nervous system speedily.

CHAPTER IV.

Diseases from Defective Nutrition

RHEUMATISM—GOUT—DIABETES—RICKETS— SCROF-
ULA.

Defective nutrition gives rise to a number of diseases that differ widely in their character, symptoms, and general effects on the system. Some of these diseases may be due primarily to defective digestion, others to imperfect assimilation or distribution of the foods already digested, while others may result simply from the lack of certain elements in the food that are necessary to supply the waste of special tissues. Under this heading are usually included rheumatism, gout, diabetes, rickets, and scrofula.

RHEUMATISM.

Rheumatism is a constitutional disease of an inflammatory character, which is due to the presence of an acid, known as lithic acid, in the blood. It attacks the joints, ligaments, or muscles, and receives various names according to the character of the disease and the parts affected. When the joints become the seat of the disease, it is spoken of as articular, and when the muscles are similarly attacked it is called muscular rheumatism. It is also divided into acute and chronic rheumatism. This latter division is the most common, and the term acute is applied to any form of the disease, which comes on quickly, with intense pain and high fever. When the disease is of long standing, and the pains, which are less severe, come on at intervals and extend over considerable time, it is said to be chronic.

The excess of lithic acid in the blood, which is the predisposing cause of rheumatism, is invariably due to imperfect digestion; and it may be safely set down as a rule that where the stomach, liver, and bowels are in a healthy condition the disease is impossible. Among the exciting causes of the disease may be mentioned exposure to cold, getting the clothing and feet wet, and the sudden checking of perspiration; but these causes will not alone produce rheumatism, unless the person is predisposed to it by the presence of acid in the system.

The usual symptoms of indigestion, with coated tongue, constipated bowels, and impaired appetite, invariably precede an attack of rheumatism. Then a tired feeling, with soreness of the muscles, darting or shooting pains in various parts of the body, and a general stiffness of the joints may be felt for some days. These symptoms are followed by a chill and the development of fever. Now the affected parts become hot, swollen, red, and very painful to the slightest motion or pressure. There is severe headache, which, together with the pains in the joints and muscles, render sleep impossible. The inflammation may begin in one joint or set of muscles, and after a day or two pass to other joints or muscles, when the local symptoms from the part first affected are considerably relieved. Thus in a week or ten days all the joints or muscles may be successively attacked, and the parts first affected may again become the seat of the disease and the pain be more severe than at first. In some cases the disease may attack the heart, which produces intense pain, and may often result fatally in a short time. The skin is hot and dry, the urine scanty and high-colored, and when perspiration does occur it is strongly acid, as is also the urine. These are the symptoms that generally manifest themselves in what is called acute or inflammatory rheumatism, or rheumatic fever, as it is sometimes called.

Chronic rheumatism is in most respects entirely different from the acute form of the disease. It usually manifests itself in the joints and is limited to those that are first attacked. Redness and swelling are less pronounced, and the pain, which is not so violent in character, is increased by motion, while any febrile symptoms that may occur are developed during damp weather. A creaking noise is heard in the joints on motion, which is due to the formation of deposits of a limy character around the articular surfaces. When muscular pains are present they are due to an inflammation that extends to the sheaths of the tendons of the muscles that are near the diseased joints; but chronic rheumatism rarely attacks the muscles alone.

Lumbago is a name popularly given to rheumatism when it is confined to the muscles of the back. Intercostal rheumatism is that form that attacks the small muscles situated between the ribs and brought into action during respiration.

Treatment.—The first consideration in the treatment of rheumatism should be to regulate the diet. In most cases it would be best to abstain from eating entirely, even for three or four days. This can be done much more easily than is usually supposed, when a person is suffering from an acute attack of rheumatism. The advantage of this course is that with the absence of food no excess of lithic acid is produced, and that already in the system is soon eliminated. When fasting is impracticable, meat diet should be avoided and the patient should be confined to fish, oysters, vegetables, and fruit; but, as before stated, the diet should be as light as possible.

Our Home Liver Pill should be given at the beginning of the disease, with a view of overcoming the torpid condition of the liver and bowels, and this should be followed by our Rheumatic Pill, which should be taken after each meal, and in severe cases two pills are required at a dose. When the inflammatory symptoms are very severe the fever may be greatly allayed by the administration of fifteen grains of the salicylate of soda, dissolved in water, every three hours. This will promote perspiration, aid in relieving the intense pain, and diminish the fever. The affected joints must be kept as quiet as possible, and warm fomentations of hops applied to them will often afford great relief to the sufferer. When the severity of the symptoms has subsided our Rheumatic Pill will be found the best remedy to eliminate the acid from the system and prevent a recurrence of the disease. In chronic rheumatism the only treatment necessary is to keep the liver and bowels in a healthy condition by the use of our Home Liver Pill and to continue our Rheumatic Pill as long as any soreness of the joints or muscles is felt.

In all cases where the joints are enlarged and the muscles remain sore after the disease has subsided, Turkish baths will be found of great benefit; but care must be taken to have the body properly cooled before leaving the bath or otherwise additional cold may be taken. The use of the galvanic current of electricity will also be found beneficial in promoting the absorption of deposits in and about the joints.

Stimulants of all kinds must be avoided during an attack of rheumatism, and persons predisposed to the disease should under all circumstances avoid wine and malt liquors. If stimulants are used at all the stronger alcoholic beverages are the most advantageous.

GOUT.

Gout is another of the constitutional diseases that depends upon the presence of an excess of lithic acid in the blood for its development. It is closely analogous to rheumatism and in fact might properly be said to be simply a variety of that disease. High living and the consequent derangements of digestion are the more common causes of the disease, although in some cases we have pronounced attacks of the gout in persons who live on very light diet; but in these cases some form of indigestion will always be found to have preceded the attack. It is claimed by many that gout is a characteristically inherited disease, but careful observation will demonstrate to the satisfaction of any observer that it is due more to the improper habits of the person than to any hereditary transmission. It usually attacks the smaller joints, as the joints of the toes, especially the great toe, and also the joints of the hands. The feet are the most common seat of the disease, and it attacks men in middle life more frequently than any other class of persons.

Acute attacks of gout resemble those of rheumatism with the exception that they are invariably confined to the place where they first began. After the joints of the feet have been affected the disease may extend to the knee and even to the hip. When the disease is once developed the attacks occur frequently, though less severe, while each attack is liable to last longer than its predecessor.

In the chronic form of the disease the joints remain permanently enlarged as a result of the limy deposits that take place. Marked deformities of the joints are thus produced.

Treatment.—Here, too, special attention must be given to the diet. Stimulants must be avoided and an entire abstinence from food insisted upon for a few days. When this is objected to, one or two severe paroxysms of gout will invariably induce the patient to try any means that is likely to effect a cure. Meats of all kinds should be withheld, and the food should be purely vegetable. The torpid liver and constipation must be relieved by Home Liver Pills taken every night, and where there is much acidity of the stomach about twenty grains of bi-carbonate of soda should be taken an hour before the liver pill. The continued use of our Rheumatic Pill will promptly relieve the worst attacks of gout when attention is given to the condition of the bowels and diet. The affected parts should be kept perfectly quiet and on a level with the body. This position prevents the settling of blood in the inflamed part and thus diminishes the severity of the pain. Hot applications and the Turkish bath are also valuable auxiliaries in the treatment of the chronic form of gout.

DIABETES.

Diabetes is a disease of defective nutrition, which is not easily recognized at first, as it is not attended by any pronounced symptoms by which the patient's attention is directed to the real nature of the trouble. It is characterized by a gradual but continued loss of flesh, a feeling of weariness, great thirst, the excessive quantity of urine passed, and finally by the presence of sugar in the urine.

It is impossible to state any special cause for this disease, nor can we say what part of the body is most affected by it. The stomach is always the starting point, and the first symptoms are those of indigestion. The liver is also torpid and enlarged, and after a time becomes fatty. The heart also takes on a condition of fatty degeneration, and the kidneys are somewhat enlarged and congested, though not as much changed as other organs.

When a general loss of flesh is noticed, with excessive urinary secretions, the urine should be examined by a competent physician, and strict attention given to whatever treatment is determined on.

Treatment.—Strict attention must be given to the diet, and any impairment in digestion must be corrected. The torpid condition of the liver and bowels must be overcome by the continued use of our Home Liver Pills, and our Dyspepsia Pills must be taken as directed after each meal.

The diet must be free from all foods containing

starch or sugar. This necessitates the exclusion of white flour bread, potatoes, corn, rice, beets, pastry, puddings, and everything containing sugar. Skimmed milk and buttermilk are both good articles of diet, but other fluids should be avoided as much as possible. Gluten bread can be used instead of ordinary bread, and meats, fish, and eggs may be freely used.

The custom of using mineral waters and medicines that act on the kidneys cannot be too severely condemned; such remedies do harm instead of good.

Fluid extract of ergot, given in thirty drop doses, in a tablespoonful of water, three or four times a day, is one of the best remedies that can be given to decrease the flow of urine and allay the thirst. Our Nerve Tonic Pill should be used when the patient feels weak and prostrated, as it will give decided tone to the nervous system, and thus restore, the general strength of the patient.

It is necessary that the mind should be free from business cares, and that the physical strength should not be exhausted by work. Moderate exercise and fresh air are essential, however, but these must be had without causing weariness, which comes on readily after slight effort.

RICKETS.

The term rickets is applied to that form of defective nutrition in which the bones of the child remain soft and flexible at a time when they should be firm and unyielding. It is characteristically a disease of childhood, and is due to some defect of nutrition by which the earthy material is supplied in insufficient quantities with the food, or the organs of nutrition are so deranged as to prevent these materials from being carried in the circulation to supply the bony structure. In such cases the flesh of the child will waste away, and the digestion is so disturbed that vomiting and diarrhea are frequently present. When the child begins to walk the weight of the body causes bending of the long bones and marked deformities of the joints. As a result we have curvature of the spine, bow legs, knock knees, and a variety of similar disorders.

Treatment.—Everything that is calculated to nourish the child and improve its general condition must be resorted to. Rich animal broth must be given to young children, and pure cow's milk, properly prepared, must be substituted for the mother's milk. Fresh air, bathing, and a sufficient supply of warm clothing are also indispensable. Scott's Emulsion of Cod Liver Oil with the hypophosphites of lime and soda should be given in tablespoonful doses three or four times a day. This remedy, being composed of some of the materials that form bony tissue, is supposed to supply these materials in quantities sufficient to produce a hardening of the bony structures.

A surgeon should be consulted in all cases of deformity.

SCROFULA.

Scrofula is usually considered a constitutional blood disease transmitted from parent to offspring, and is supposed to be one of the constitutional transmitted taints resulting from syphilis. Many physicians apply the name to a great variety of disorders, and it is a convenient term to use when they do not know what the real nature of the trouble is. The time was when all diseases of the bones, glands, and skin were considered to be scrofulous in character, but more recent investigation has demonstrated that all these disorders are due to direct predisposing and exciting causes.

The condition that is generally recognized as scrofula is one where there is an enlargement of the glands of the neck and other portions of the body which may extend to suppuration and the discharge of matter. This condition is invariably due to some cause of defective nutrition where the effete material of the system is not properly thrown off, and is thus accumulated in the glands whose special office it is to remove the waste material. After the accumulation has continued so long as to enlarge these glands, nature makes an effort to throw off this waste material, and as a result we have inflammation and breaking down of the glands and the formation of matter, which is discharged, and thus the system is freed from an unhealthy condition; and the process by which this is done is spoken of as scrofula. Persons suffering from this peculiar condition usually have a sallow or white condition of skin, flabby muscles, and a general appearance of feebleness and lack of vital power. Any wound or bruise heals with difficulty, and glandular enlargements are developed upon the slightest exposure to cold.

Treatment.—Nutritious food which should include plenty of rare beef and mutton, must always be given to this class of patients; moderate but regular exercise should be employed, and frequent bathing is essential to keep up the action of the skin. Ten drops of dyalized iron given in a teaspoonful of water three or four times a day will also be found to serve an admirable purpose.

With a view of promoting the action of the lymphatic glands and thus enabling them to throw off the effete material that has accumulated in the system, our Alterative Pill should be given as directed and continued until a decided improvement is manifest in the patient. As these conditions more often occur before the age of fourteen or fifteen it is important to watch the health of the child until after that period, when a complete change usually takes place and the symptoms of the so-called scrofula then often disappear. Similar disorders occur later in life, and although attributed to scrofula are often due to other causes and require such treatment as may be found valuable for the removal of the exciting causes in each individual case.

CHAPTER V.

Specific Blood Diseases.

SYPHILIS—HYDROPHOBIA—GLANDERS.

Under the head of Specific Blood Diseases are included such as are produced by local inoculation of some specific poison, which enters the system, and after variable periods of time, ranging from two weeks to three months, develops constitutional symptoms that are characteristic of the spécial pioson introduced. Syphilis, hydrophobia, and glanders, are the principal diseases of this class.

SYPHILIS.

Syphilis is a constitutional blood disease which originates from impure coitus. It first appears as a local sore on the genitals, and is called a chancre. The poison from this sore is soon absorbed into the system and poisons the blood, thus giving rise to a variety of eruptions on the skin and mucous surfaces, which are spoken of as secondary or constitutional syphilis.

A full description of the symptoms and complications of this disease cannot be given in a popular work of this character, but those desirous of understanding the nature and treatment of this disease should send for " The Health of Men," a book devoted to the physiological functions and the diseases of the male organs.*

Persons suffering from this disease should give it immediate attention on the first appearance of the local sore, with a view to preventing it from entering the blood and thus becoming constitutional. If a physician cannot be consulted, our Alterative Pill should be taken at once and continued regularly for two or three months, as in this way only can a person be safe against serious secondary disorders that develop after syphilis becomes constitutional. Full directions for local treatment and the treatment of the various secondary conditions will be found in the work referred to in the foot note.

HYDROPHOBIA.

Hydrophobia is the name given a disease developed in man by the inoculation of poisonous saliva introduced by the bite of a rabid dog. The disease is not as common as is usually supposed, for many of the conditions believed to be rabies in the dog are entirely different in character, and the

---

* This volume is written by a well-known Physician and Surgeon, and published by the HOME TREATMENT COMPANY, New York. Price, $1.00.

fear of having the disease often produces a chain of nervous symptoms that closely resemble those of genuine hydrophobia. The word "hydrophobia" means "fear of water," and was first given to the disease because it was supposed that persons afflicted by it, as well as rabid dogs, had a dread of water. Recent observations, however, have shown this to be incorrect, but it is true that persons thus affected find themselves unable to swallow fluids, and consequently will refuse to take them.

The wound made by the bite of a rabid dog usually heals kindly, but after six or seven weeks, or sometimes longer, a feeling of uneasiness, loss of appetite, flashes of heat with alternating chills, sore throat, nausea and vomiting, headache and general nervous excitement, begin to show themselves. The scar becomes red and painful, and a feeling of itching and irritation is felt extending from it along the course of the nerves. These symptoms may last for a few hours or for eight or ten days, after which there is a stiffness of the muscles of the jaw and throat. It becomes difficult or impossible to swallow and every attempt to do so produces severe paroxysms of pain. Usually the spasms affect the muscles of the wind pipe, causing a hurried respiration, while the hurried expulsion of the air causes a sound somewhat resembling the bark of a dog. The mouth becomes dry, and the saliva is so thickened that all efforts to remove it by hawking increase the barking noise. After a time the nervous system becomes exhausted, there is a loss of memory and delirium, and a general condition of paralysis develops. The pupils are large, the mouth is open, and the saliva runs from the mouth or passes into the back part of the throat, causing a gurgling and choking noise, and death takes place from exhaustion or suffocation. These are the symptoms that are present in a true case of hydrophobia, but they are fortunately very rare.

In some cases, where a person has been bitten by a dog, the scar remains unchanged, and similar symptoms to those above given occur even a week or two after the bite, or may not appear for six months or more. All such cases may be set down as caused by fear, and in no way connected with the presence of rabies.

Treatment.—So far as is now known, the only treatment to be adopted is the preventive one. As soon as a person has been bitten by a dog supposed to be rabid, the wound should be applied immediately to the mouth and sucked freely until a physician can be reached, who will apply some caustic so thoroughly as to penetrate the deepest part of the wound. The galvanic cautery is also used for destroying and removing the tissue immediately around the wound. These methods prevent the poison from getting into the system, and then all possibility of hydrophobia developing is averted.

The inoculations practiced by Pasteur of Paris have proved a lamentable failure, and no reliance should be placed in them. More careful study of the nature of rabies in the dog will be a great preventive of the development of the nervous condition resembling the symptoms of hydrophobia. Such symptoms may extend to such a degree as to produce sufficient disturbance of the base of the brain and nervous system generally to cause death even when no hydrophobia is present.

GLANDERS.

Glanders is a disease affecting the glands of the mouth and the mucous membrane of the nose in horses, and is often communicated to man, and then from one individual to another. A person who has been attending to a horse suffering from glanders and soon after complains of a general languor, with pain in the back, arms, and legs, which are soon followed by chills, with flashes of heat, stiffness and soreness of the joints, impaired appetite, irritable stomach, constipated bowels, and sleeplessness, certainly has reason to suspect that he has contracted the disease. After these symptoms have developed they continue from thirty-six to forty-eight hours, when a severe chill occurs, which is immediately followed by violent fever and profuse perspiration, resembling an attack of ague and fever. The pulse is irregular and quick, the tongue parched and covered with a brown coating, the lining membrane of the nose is much inflamed, and a free, fetid discharge is developed. Great prostration occurs, and an offensive odor similar to that coming from a glandered horse is apparent about the patient The disease, if not recognized early, is apt to prove fatal in periods ranging from one to three weeks.

Treatment.—Preventive measures are of the first importance. Persons caring for horses suffering from this disease should be careful not to expose cuts or sores to contact with the saliva of the animai, and care should be taken not to allow the animal to breathe in the face. As soon as the diseased animal is attended to, the hands should be thoroughly cleansed, and the attendant snould use a solution of carbolic acid to snuff up the nostrils and gargle the throat. For this purpose put twenty drops of carbolic acid into a gobletful of tepid water; stir it up and use freely to snuff into the nose and as a gargle. Should the first symptoms be recognized, ten-grain doses of quinine should be taken every three or four hours until sixty grains are used, and about two tablespoonfuls of good whisky at about the same intervals will also prove valuable. Nutritious diet, good ventilation, and absolute quiet are necessary to ward off the disease. When it is once fully developed, however, there is very little hope of saving the patient.

CHAPTER VI.

Disease of Lungs and Air Passages

CONSUMPTION—ACUTE BRONCHITIS-CHRONIC BRON-
CHITIS — ASTHMA—ACUTE NASAL CATARRH —
ULCERATION OF THE NOSE—SORE THROAT—
QUINSY—CROUP—LOSS OF VOICE—INFLAMMA-
TION OF LARYNX—CHRONIC CATARRH—PNEU-
MONIA—PLURISY.

Under the head of Disease of the Lungs and Air-
passages are included a large number of acute inflammatory diseases that require the closest attention
of the family physician in their treatment. In such
cases it would be useless to give any general outlines
of the treatment that might be used at home, as va-
rions complications are constantly arising that must
be specially treated as they present themselves, and
such conditions can only be recognized by a person
who has had experience in the management of such
diseases. Among the diseases of this character are
included pleurisy, dropsy of the chest, pneumonia,
and acute bronchitis. The chronic diseases of the
lungs and air passages may be more satisfactorily

managed by home treatment, and we will, therefore, confine our attention to those, the most important of which are consumption, chronic bronchitis, asthma, croup, and catarrh.

CONSUMPTION.

Consumption is a popular name given to disease of the lung tissues which is characterized by a filling up of the substance of the lung by the deposit of effete material and the breaking down of the lung tissues. The deposits vary in character in different persons, and are professionally recognized as different forms of consumption. For popular consideration, however, it is unnecessary to create confusion in the mind of the reader by describing the peculiar character of the deposit which is present in the several forms of the disease.

This disease is generally considered to be inherited, but a close study of the history of consumption and the history of families will often reveal the fact that persons of the same family who have continued to live in the same locality, eat the same food, and be surrounded by the same general influences, have all suffered from the disease, but where members of that family have removed to different parts of the country and completely changed their environments they have been known to escape entirely. In fact this is true to so great an extent that it may be safely laid down as a rule that when consumption shows itself in the different members of the same family it is best under all circumstances that a change of residence should be sought at once, and in making such change attention should be given to the atmospheric conditions that are most favorable for persons predisposed to consumption. It is also well known that many persons, after having been exposed to repeated colds, even though no history of an hereditary transmission of the disease can be obtained, fall victims to it, and die in a few weeks. Such cases are often popularly called " quick consumption."

The first symptoms of the disease may be those of an ordinary cold, such as a slight cough, dry expectoration, loss of appetite, indigestion, and finally a loss of flesh and strength. In some cases there may be a general falling away of the patient without any appearance of cough. Persons thus affected, who are tall, thin, and narrow chested, should take warning at once, and either by treatment or change of climate try to avert the approaching disease. When a cough is present it is dry and sharp, more troublesome at night than during the day, and is attended with pains in the chest, shortness of breath, slight tendency to fever toward the latter part of the afternoon, and night sweats. In the first stage of the disease a free bleeding from the lungs will frequently take place. Instead of this occasioning alarm however, it should have the opposite effect, as it is an effort of nature to throw off what would otherwise become a tubercular deposit on the lungs. After such a bleeding the previous premonitory symptoms may be materially relieved for a considerable length of time. After the cough has continued for some time there is more or less expectoration, which soon assumes the character of purulent matter, and as the disease advances it will be found to sink in water. Great prostration of the system is now apparent and the appetite is entirely gone; the fever becomes more pronounced and the night sweats more prolonged, so as to often continne during the night. As the disease advances the cough becomes so troublesome and painful that sleep is almost impossible, and the expectoration changes until it assumes a greenish-yellow color, which is significant of the breaking down of the lung tissue. The voice and cough become hollow, there is a hectic flush on the cheeks, and the general prostration is so great that the patient can hardly stand.

Further description of this distressing disease is unnecessary, as the symptoms are so pronounced that no one can be mistaken as to the character of the disease.

Treatment.—The treatment of consumption is more especially applicable to the early stages. Every effort should be made to fill the lungs by inhaling as much air without stopping as possible. In this way more oxygen is taken into the lungs and the oxygen removes the effete material that would otherwise be deposited in the tissue. A change of climate is always desirable in the early stages of consumption, and it should be borne in mind that if a change is delayed until the lungs are seriously involved, the patient is better off to remain at home. In the earlier stages of the disease the climate of Colorado, Northern California, or Minnesota, is best in consequence of the rare condition of the atmosphere and the excessive oxygen, but when the disease is once developed and the cough is aggravated by a cold dry atmosphere Southern California, Georgia, and Florida, are preferable locations for consumptives.

If it were possible for a person to live in an atmosphere containing an extra amount of oxygen, the disease might be prevented entirely, or very materially delayed in its progress; but as this is impossible we are obliged to resort to such remedies as will keep up the nutrition of the body by supplying new material in excess of the waste. For this purpose Scott's Emulsion will be found to serve the best purpose. It is a preparation of Cod-liver Oil with the hypophosphites of lime and soda, and is palatable to the taste, and supplies the system with the elements necessary to build up lung tissue and maintain the strength of the patient. When taken according to directions it improves the appetite, relieves the cough, diminishes the expectoration and stops the night sweats so common in this disease.

In the way of diet, milk, cream, nutritious

meats, with plenty of fat, and good whisky, are essential to keeping up the vitality of the patient. The best nutri nent that can be used is Bovinine, which is simply beef blood, drawn from the living animal and hermetically sealed. It contains all the nutritious elements of the system in a form that can be easily assimilated by the most delicate stomach.

With a view of allaying the irritation of the throat and bronchial tubes resulting from cough, our Improved Inhaler can be used with Inhalent No. 1 several times a day. This favorable result, however, can only be expected where the case is taken in time and the treatment followed until the unfavorable symptoms disappear.

ACUTE BRONCHITIS.

Acute Bronchitis is a recent and active inflammation of the mucous membrane of the bronchial tubes. It is produced by exposure to cold and sudden changes of temperature. It is more common during the damp, changeable weather of the spring and fall, and those whose systems are debilitated from any cause are more liable to it than those of strong, robust constitutions. It is also caused by the inhalation of particles of dust from the atmosphere, or irritating gasses or vapors. The modern theory is that this disease is always caused by a specific bacillus, or disease germ.

The condition popularly called a "cold in the chest," is a mild form of acute bronchitis.

The symptoms of this disease are a dry, harsh cough, a sense of rawness of the throat and bronchial tubes, followed by languor, chills, and flashes of heat. The throat becomes constricted, pain is felt when a long breath is taken, there is marked hoarseness, and glarry mucus is brought up by the cough. After a few days the expectoration increases and is easily raised, and becomes yellowish in color, and purulent in character. When free expectoration is established the pain and soreness decrease, and the fever disappears. A mild case lasts from ten to twenty days, but in severe cases the symptoms are more aggravated, and may last for several weeks.

Treatment.—At the beginning of the disease a hot lemonade or whisky sling may be given to cause free perspiration. To allay the fever ten drops of tincture of aconite root may be put in eight tablespoonfuls of water, and of this a teaspoonful should be taken every half hour until the fever subsides.

Our Inhalent No. 1 can then be used in our Improved Inhaler.

CHRONIC BRONCHITIS.

By Chronic Bronchitis is meant a chronic inflammation of the larger air tubes that ramify through the lungs, which are called bronchial tubes. This disease may be dependent upon some disorder of the heart or lungs, and is often associated with Bright's disease, and is also one of the prominent symptoms of infectious diseases. Sometimes it is the result of a frequent recurrence of colds affecting the bronchial tubes, which finally become chronically inflamed, and the inflammation may even extend to ulceration.

Among the more prominent symptoms are frequent paroxysms of coughing, the sticky character of the expectoration, difficulty of breathing, with more or less wheezing during respiration. In severe cases many of the symptoms may resemble consumption, but there is not the extreme emaciation, nor the purulent and heavy character of the expectoration. Bleeding from the bronchial tubes may sometimes take place, but when it does the blood is dark and not likely to form clots, while in consumption the blood is of a bright scarlet color.

Treatment.—The treatment of chronic bronchitis will depend very much upon the severity of the disease and the constitution of the patient. As there is often extreme thickness of the lining membrane of the tubes, some alterative medicine will be required in most cases. Our Home Alterative Pill will be found of great benefit, and our Improved Inhaler, with Inhalent No. 1, will be found to give decided relief, and in many cases to effect a radical cure. The free use of Scott's Emulsion is desirable. It must always be borne in mind, however, that the summer season is the best time of the year for the treatment of all bronchial troubles. In the

severer forms of the disease the inflammation extends to ulceration of the mucous surfaces. When
this condition develops the expectoration has the
characteristics of ordinary pus, and there is generally more or less constitutional fever and general
prostration. Rich cream, whisky, and a generally
nutritious diet, must be resorted to in all such
cases.

ASTHMA.

The term Asthma is applied to a spasmodic difficulty of breathing, which usually comes on suddenly, and after continuing for a variable length of
time will disappear, leaving the patient, to all ap-
pearances, free from any diseased condition of the
organs of breathing. The true nature of the disease is not well understood, but is claimed by many
to be of a nervous character, and to be developed
from sudden irritation extending to the nerves that
supply the mucous surface of the air passages and
control the muscles of breathing. When an attack
takes place it is apt to come on again without much
warning, and many people suffer for years, especially in certain localities, without being able to get
a moment's relief.

The first attack of asthma begins with an ordinary cold in the head, with slight bronchial irritation,
headache, and a feeling of general depression. It
is likely to occur any hour in the twenty-four, but
usually takes place at night. The most important

symptom of an asthmatic attack. is the distress that follows every attempt to inhale air into the lungs, and it will sometimes seem that the more effort a person makes to breathe the more difficult it is to do so. With every breath that passes the windpipe there is a loud wheezing, the face becomes flushed and even assumes a bluish tinge, the body is bathed in cold perspiration, the eyeballs seem to protrude, the eyes stare, the muscles of the neck become fixed, the lips parched and the patient can hardly gasp. A paroxysm may last only a few minutes or may continue for several hours without intermission. When the paroxysm is over a person may go a day, several days, or many weeks without a recurrence, while it frequently happens that an attack comes on suddenly, when a person goes from one locality to another to stay for a few days. We have known of persons who would be entirely free from asthma in New York City and Cairo, Egypt, but could not live in any place else without having several attacks during the course of a week.

Treatment.—The first thing to consider in the treatment of asthma is to relieve the impending or existing paroxysm. The simplest means of doing this, which can always be procured within a short time, is to burn dry stramonium leaves or nitre paper, and to inhale the smoke as it escapes from the burning mass. The nitre paper is prepared by steeping ordinary blotting paper in a strong solution of saltpetre, and then allowing it to dry so that the water is driven off and the saltpetre remains in the tissue of the paper. Our Improved Inhaler, with our asthmatic inhalation, will be found more convenient and more effective as an inhalation during the paroxysm than anything that has heretofore been offered to the public. With a view to relieving the spasmodic condition of the muscles of respiration, and to give the patient relief during the night, our Neurodine Tablet should be taken as directed at bedtime, when a comfortable night's rest can always be insured. After the paroxysm of asthma has passed, the continued use of our Inhaler, and the administration of one Neurodine Tablet on going to bed, will often relieve the spasmodic conditions that tend to produce the paroxysms, and have in many cases effected what appears to be a radical cure of asthma.

ACUTE NASAL CATARRH.

When the mucous membrane of the nose is attacked by an acute inflammation it is called a cold in the head, coryza, or acute nasal catarrh. It is due to exposure to cold, sudden changes of temperature, going from a warm room out-doors when overheated, wet feet, or the inhalation of any irritating gas or vapor through the nose.

An attack of this kind is usually attended by muscular soreness, general languor, headache, and chilliness, a dryness of the nose, inclination to sneeze, and an inability to breathe through the nose when the mouth is closed. A profuse watery discharge soon takes place from the nostrils, which gradually becomes thick and offensive. The sense of smell is diminished or destroyed, the voice assumes a nasal twang and the mouth must be kept open in order to breathe. During the fall, winter, and spring months persons are very liable to this form of cold and may have repeated attacks at short intervals during the changeable weather. In this manner the membranes become thickened and a condition of chronic nasal catarrh is produced.

Treatment.—With the first symptoms of a cold in the head the feet should be soaked in mustard water as hot as can be borne before retiring to bed, and a hot lemonade or whisky sling should be administered, while plenty of bed-clothing should be used to retain the warmth of the body. This will often result in a free perspiration and the patient awakens in the morning without the least symptom of the disease. When attainable a Turkish bath taken at the beginning of an attack will invariably break it up and save the patient much annoyance. Should the symptoms continue the second day, our Malaria Pill should be used as directed for a day or two, and tincture of aconite may be given in one-drop doses, every half hour whenever the skin feels hot and feverish.

For local treatment our Improved Home Inhaler should be used several times a day with Inhalent No. 1, and persons who are liable to frequent attacks of cold in the head should use it regularly whenever they feel the first symptoms of a fresh cold.

ULCERATION OF THE NOSE.

Persons who are weak and debilitated from any cause or whose blood is impoverished are liable to suffer from ulceration of the mucous membrane as well as of the bones of the nose after frequent attacks of acute catarrh.

The first symptoms are those to be hereafter described under the heading of chronic catarrh, but soon the discharges become very offensive and after a time small pieces of bone will be found to be mixed with them. The first indication of this should warn the patient of the extensive destruction of bone that is liable to follow, and an experienced surgeon should be consulted without delay.*

SORE THROAT.

The mucous membrane of the large cavity forming the back part of the throat, which is called the pharynx, the tonsils, and the soft palate, are frequently affected by acute inflammation resulting from cold, and while different names are given to the inflammation affecting these several tissues, the general term of sore throat is commonly applied to one or all, from the fact that there is tenderness

---

* We shall always be glad to recommend experienced surgeons to any one writing us for information,

of the throat and pain with every attempt at swallowing, when these parts are inflamed.

There is a general feeling of dryness and obstruction in the throat, the membrane is swollen and very red, the soft palate is thickened and elongated, and often the tonsils are so enlarged as to fill up the entire throat. Sometimes the tonsils are covered with ulcerated patches, which indicates a severer form of inflammation. These patches are isolated at first and must not be mistaken for the extensive ulceration characteristic of diphtheria. Many physicians pronounce every case of this kind "diphtheria," and then take the credit of speedily curing that disease.

Treatment.—In all cases of sore throat the voice should be used as little as possible. Mustard plasters may be applied externally over the seat of the soreness and left on until the skin is decidedly red. This draws the blood to the surface and relieves the local inflammation of the throat. For the local treatment our Improved Inhaler should be used with Inhalent No. 1, as often as the soreness and dryness of the parts become annoying to the patient.

QUINSY.

The two little glands generally called the tonsils, situated on either side of the throat, between the folds of the mucous membrane, are sometimes the seat of a local inflammation that does not extend to other parts. It is due to exposure to cold or damp, or any causes that tend to produce inflammation of any of these tissues. This inflammation is spoken of as tonsillitis, but it often receives the common name quinsy, though, properly speaking, the name quinsy should not be applied unless suppuration takes place and matter forms in the interior of the tonsils.

The symptoms are the same as those described for sore throat, but when matter forms in the tonsil, a deep seated, throbbing pain is felt sometimes for several days, and every attempt to swallow is followed by the most excruciating suffering. In some cases even the breathing becomes very difficult, in consequence of the filling up of the cavity of the throat. This severe pain, especially that of the deep-seated throbbing character, indicates the formation of matter.

Treatment.—On the start the same treatment as recommended for general sore throat should be followed, but when the tonsils seem to be very large, and the pain above mentioned is suddenly developed, the best course to pursue is to have the tonsils lanced by a physician, even if no matter be present. This allows a large quantity of blood to escape and thus relieves the congestion of the part so that in many instances the matter will not form afterwards. Where this cannot be done, hot fomentations of hops, or flaxseed meal poultices, should be applied to the throat so as to favor the speedy formation of the matter and a spontaneous discharge of the same, for no relief can be obtained until the local distention is relieved in cne of these ways. For the relief of the intense suffering our Neurodine Tablet may be given as directed. After the pus has discharged, the Improved Inhaler with Inhalent No. 1, should be used two or three times a day till the soreness entirely disappears.

CROUPS.

The mucous, or lining membrane of the larynx (upper part of the windpipe) in children is liable to be affected by an inflammation to which the common name croup has been applied. There are three varieties of the disease, which are named respectively mucous, spasmodic, and membranous croup. Mucous Croup is a mild inflammation of the membrane resulting from cold. It comes on suddenly during the night, with difficult breathing and a croupy cough which awakens the child even out of a sound sleep. Sometimes a slight cough with the usual symptoms of cold may be present during the day, but nothing is thought of it. A rough, whistling sound accompanies the breathing, the cry and voice are hoarse and the cough has a rough metallic sound. Mucus accumulates in the throat, and renders the breathing difficult and even causes symptoms of strangulation. The cough of croup when once heard can easily be recognized by any one, while the rattling of the mucus readily distinguishes this from the other varieties of croup.

At first the skin is hot and dry, and the pulse full and hard, but soon the extremities become cold, the skin is covered with a cold perspiration and the pulse becomes rapid and feeble.

Spasmodic Croup is also due to cold, but the attacks are not severe and are soon over. A slight hoarseness and cough in the evening is followed by a few hours of restless sleep from which the child awakes with a paroxysm of difficult breathing. A hoarse, metallic cough next occurs, while the child cannot speak above a whisper. There is no fever or other constitutional disturbance, and no accumulation of mucus in the throat; and in a few minutes the paroxysm ceases, and the child speedily falls a sleep again. After an interval of a few minutes another paroxysm occurs, and so they may continue during the night, but in the morning there is no symptom of the trouble left, excepting possibly a slight cough.

Membranous Croup begins as an ordinary cold and gradually increases for several days before the croupy symptoms come on. A tough, tenacious mucus collects in the windpipe, which causes a whistling kind of breathing, with spasmodic attacks of croupy cough. The skin is dry and hot, and the pulse rapid and hard, the breathing is permanently difficult, while the croupy cough comes on at intervals. If these symptoms are not relieved before the mucus in the windpipe obstructs the breathing the skin and lips assume a purple hue, the extrem-

ities become cold, and languor and stupor soon follow, because enough air does not reach the lungs
to supply the blood with the oxygen necessary to
sustain life.

Treatment.—Hot fomentations of hops should be
applied around the throat, and changed every half
hour so as to keep up the heat, and when the skin
is hot and dry the following should be administered:
Tincture of aconite root, ten drops; tincture of lobelia, thirty drops; water, eight tablespoonfuls.
Dose, a teaspoonful every fifteen or twenty minutes. In cases of spasmodic croup a teaspoonful of
tincture of gelsemium may be substituted for the
ten drops of tincture of aconite in the above. In
severe cases, where the breathing becomes greatly
obstructed, it is essential to cause vomiting so as to
dislodge the accumulating false membrane before
it completely obstructs the breathing. For this
purpose twenty drops of tincture of lobelia with ten
drops of tincture of ipecac should be given in a
tablespoonful of sweetened water, every fifteen or
twenty minutes till vomiting is produced. After
the vomiting the child is very much prostrated, but
if the phlegm has been thrown off reaction will
soon take place.

Great relief is often obtained by pouring boiling vinegar upon a handful of hops, in a tea-
pot, and allowing the child to inhale the steam
from the spout for ten or fifteen minutes at a
time.

LOSS OF VOICE.

A complete Loss of Voice will sometimes follow a cold in the throat and windpipe, and it is often unattended by pain. It is due to a relaxation of the vocal cords, and to effect a cure all attempts at talking must be avoided.

Treatment.—Our Nerve Tonic Pill must be used to give the requisite tone to the relaxed condition of the throat, and for local treatment our Improved Inhaler, with Inhalent No. 1, should be used every hour or two during the day.

INFLAMMATION OF THE LARYNX.

The upper part of the windpipe is technically called the larynx and the lower part is called the trachea, while the branches that extend to the lungs and their several ramifications are called bronchial tubes. The larynx is often the seat of an inflammation, either acute or chronic, which may have been an extension of an inflammation of the back part of the throat, or may have been produced primarily by cold or sudden changes of temperature, as well as by the inhalation of irritating gases. The inflammation of these air passages is usually spoken of as a cold on the chest; and this name is not inappropriate when any of the mucous surfaces of the air passages below the pharynx become inflamed. The symptoms attending upon the inflammation of these surfaces are a sense of dryness and a desire to clear the throat, a sharp pain on swallowing, soreness and stiffness of the neck over the windpipe, a harsh, dry cough with a scraping or raw sensation of the surfaces, a frothy mucus expectoration which gradually changes its character and presents a yellowish appearance as if mixed with pus, while more or less hoarseness is present, and in some cases there is a complete loss of voice. These symptoms may last but a few days, or may continue for weeks, or even result in a chronic inflammation of the part affected.

Treatment.—It is wise in all such cases to avoid exposure to cold or damp air and avoid using the voice as much as possible. A mustard plaster should be placed over the seat of the pain, on the neck and upper part of the chest. The hot mustard footbath is always serviceable in the onset of the disease, and a hot lemonade or hot whisky sling taken at bed-time will often relieve the local inflammation. Our Improved Inhaler with Inhalent No. 1, should be used to secure relief of the local symptoms, for this is one of the few instruments that will admit of a medicated air being carried directly to the air passages, so as to reach the inflamed surfaces. Home Cough Lozenges should be taken as directed every hour or two to promote expectoration and relieve the patient of coughing. Even children over a year old can take about one-quarter of a lozenge every couple of hours, if necessary.

CHRONIC CATARRH.

By Chronic Catarrh in this connection we mean a chronic inflammation of the mucous surfaces of the air passages of the head and throat, although the term is also applied, as already stated, to inflammation of similar surfaces in other portions of the body. The acute inflammation just described, especially when it occurs frequently, often leaves the membrane in a weakened and inflamed condition. It matters little where the inflammation starts, when it begins to assume a chronic form it usually spreads along the continuous surfaces until it reaches the membrane of the nose. The cavities in the head, above the nose and back of the throat, become involved in one continuous condition of chronic inflammation. When this condition is once developed the membranes may be dry and hot, but more commonly a thick tenacious mucus is continually being secreted from the inflamed surfaces. Usually the secretion accumulates in the back of the throat, and forms hard lumps during the night, which the patient finds it difficult to dislodge by repeated hawking and coughing during the morning. This constant effort to clear the throat of the accumulated mucus aggravates the trouble, makes the voice rough and husky, and occasions a continuous hacking cough. In severe cases there is a constant pain above the nose and across the eyebrows, an offensive odor to the breath, and in many cases a complete loss of the sense of smell. So severe are these symptoms during the cold weather that every effort to treat the disease is liable to be followed by repeated fresh colds and an aggravation of the symptoms, so that persons suffering from catarrh usually think the disease cannot be cured. We have found out by long experience, however, that, when properly treated during the summer months, the worst cases of catarrh can be radically cured, and it was by efforts in this direction that led to the introduction of our simple Improved In haler, the use of which, with our Inhalent No. 1, if persistently followed during the summer, will cure the worst cases of chronic catarrh. It may, however, often be necessary to resort to our Alterative Pill for the purpose of reducing the extreme thickness of the mucous membrane which has been developed by the long continuance of the disease. This improves the condition of the blood and materially aids the local treatment in affecting the radical cure.

Some cases may require the application of strong medicines to the affected surface for a few weeks before the home treatment can do any good. These applications, however, should only be made by an experienced physician. It is useless, however, to begin the treatment of such cases during the winter months. We are prepared to give patients from the country the most skillful treatment, with home comforts, while in the city.

PNEUMONIA.

Pneumonia is an inflammation of the lung tissues proper. It is also called "lung fever," and "winter fever." It is produced by exposure to cold, and attacks those whose vitality has been reduced from any cause. Some claim that it is due to a disease germ, or pneumonia bacillus.

A general depression or languor, a hacking cough, quick-short breathing, a sense of oppression in the chest, with chilliness and coldness of the extremities are the early symptoms. These may be felt for a day or two, when a decided chill comes on which may last for one or two hours. As soon as the chill passes febrile symptoms come on, and the respiration becomes shorter, and the breathing difficult.

Whenever these symptoms manifest themselves a physician should be sent for without delay, and till he arrives an effort should be made to promote perspiration. In short a free perspiration must be maintained throughout the disease, and the pulse and temperature must be kept down with tincture of veratrum viride in two or three drop doses, every half hour, till the skin becomes moist or slight nausea is produced. But no one should attempt to treat this disease without the aid of a physician.

PLEURISY.

Pleurisy is an inflammation of a membrane called the pleura, which lines the inner surface of the walls of the thorax and incases the lungs. The pleura may be the primary seat of the inflammation, or the disease may extend to it from the lungs. It begins with a chill, fever, pain in the side, and difficult breathing. After a time the pain is intense with every full breath, and is of a sharp, cutting character.

This is also a disease that should not be treated without the aid of a physician, as many serious complications are liable to follow it, if not properly treated from the start.

CHAPTER VII.

Diseases of the Nervous System.

HEADACHE —VERTIGO — SPINAL IRRITATION—CON-
VULSIONS—EPILEPSY—ST. VITUS DANCE—HYS-
TERIA —HICCOUGH—SEA SICKNESS— NEURAL-
GIA—PARALYSIS.

Diseases of the nervous system include all affec-
tions of the brain, spinal cord, nerves of special sense
and the nerves of motion and sensation. Each of
these are liable to diseases both acute and chronic
in character, but many of them are so important
and serious in their nature as to require the attention of the physician, so that each symptom may be
properly managed as it develops. Among these
acute disorders are congestion and inflammation of
the brain, apoplexy, spinal meningitis, convulsions,
lockjaw, and insanity, from whatever local condition it may arise. Among the nervous disorders
that may be treated at home must be mentioned
headache, vertigo, spinal irritation, epilepsy, hysteria, St. Vitus dance, hiccough, delirium tremens,
neuralgia of all kinds, toothache, sunstroke, and
some forms of paralysis.

HEADACHE.

Headache is generally looked upon as of little significance, and many persons allow themselves to be sufferers from some of its forms for years, without doing anything in the way of medical treatment. This is a mistake, and it should be borne in mind that severe headaches, frequently recurring, often result in more serious disorders of the brain. There are many forms of headache, each of which is due to a variety of causes, though it may often be a symptom of some other disease.

The principal forms of headache are the nervous, bilious, congestive, plethoric, and sick headache; while we also have rheumatic headache, renal headache, and headache resulting from organic changes in the brain itself, which is usually called organic headache. It is needless to say that all these headaches are attended with severe pain in the head, which many times become almost unbearable.

Nervous headache is more liable to attack persons of an excitable nervous disposition, and is more common in women than in men. Among the existing causes of this form of headache may be mentioned excessive mental effort, business worry, loss of sleep, sexual excess, diseases of the womb, etc.

In bilious headache the skin is sallow, the bowels constipated, and there is a general feeling of depression present. The pain is confined to the eyebrows and forehead, and is of a throbbing character. The skin is hot, the muscles are sore, the tongue is coated, the appetite poor, and nausea is usually present, though vomiting rarely occurs.

Sick headache is invariably due to some derangement of the digestion. A dull heavy pain is felt upon waking or soon after getting up, the usual symptoms of indigestion are present, and continuous nausea followed by vomiting invariably manifests itself. Every attempt to move increases the nausea, and the vomiting rarely subsides until the contents of the stomach, with considerable bile, have been thrown up. The pain often locates itself on one side, most commonly the left, and will be felt frequently darting through the ball of the eye.

Plethoric headache is a form that usually attacks persons who are full-blooded. The symptoms are extreme fullness and throbbing through the temples and over the eyebrows, dizziness following the slightest motion, frequent bleeding from the nose, and sometimes diarrhea, and the pain is of a pulsating, throbbing character.

The rheumatic headache attacks persons suffering from rheumatism. It is felt more in the back of the head and is of a dull aching character, without throbbing. The affected part is tender on pressure and the skin of the forehead and scalp is cool and moist. The pain is worse toward evening and is more severe as the acute symptoms of rheumatism diminish.

In some conditions of the system where there is an accumulation of oxalate of lime in the urine with a scanty flow of that secretion, and in all disorders of the kidneys, a feeling of soreness is felt at the base of the brain, which extends upward from the sides and centers itself on the top of the head.

In congestion or inflammation of the brain or the membranes covering it, headache is a prominent symptom, but the other acute symptoms are of such a character as to indicate positively the nature of the trouble, and the headache is consequently of secondary importance.

Treatment.—The condition of the stomach and bowels must always be considered in every case of headache, as constipation and indigestion will invariably aggravate and often indirectly produce the several headaches above described. It is, therefore, advisable for all persons thus afflicted to keep the liver and bowels regular by the use of our Home Liver Pills, and where the digestion is impaired our Dyspepsia Pill should be used regularly until digestion is properly performed. In the bilious, sick, and plethoric headaches, this treatment is of the greatest importance, and must be followed up regularly if a cure is desired. Nervous headache also requires hygienic consideration. Excessive mental labor must be avoided, and the nervous system toned up by the use of proper remedies. In women, where the headache may be due to some uterine disorder, that condition should be looked

after before permanent relief can be obtained.
With a view to giving general tone to the nervous
system our Nerve Tonic Pill will be found specially
serviceable.   Soaking the feet in hot water before
retiring, and taking a hot lemonade or whisky
sling, containing about an ounce of good whisky,
will often relieve a severe headache.   This is particularly true in cases of sick or bilious headache,
Where the bowels have been constipated in the
morning a full dose (one ounce) of Rochelle salts
taken before breakfast will move the bowels in a
short time, and in that way the headache will often
be relieved.   In the rheumatic or renal headache,
the disease of which the headache is a symptom
must be specially treated as indicated under the
respective headings. With a view to giving prompt
relief from any severe headache, nothing is better
than our Neurodine Tablet.   If taken according to
directions it will stop the pain by relieving the congestion of the nerve centers, thereby producing a
natural sleep.   In nervous headaches this pill
should be given every night at bedtime so as to
quiet the patient and permit a natural sleep, and
the Nerve Tonic Pill should be given during the
day for the purpose of toning up the general system.   In a few cases of headache from indigestion,
where the stomach is evidently disturbed by the
presence of undigested food, an emetic may be
given with advantage.   The simplest thing for this
purpose is warm water and salt, or mustard water.

After the stomach is thus emptied an ounce of good whisky or brandy will often give prompt relief.

VERTIGO.

Vertigo, or dizziness, is not of itself a disease, but a symptom which attends many other disorders. Diseases of the heart, stomach, and ear, are often attended by it. It is also frequently present in women undergoing "change of life."

Treatment.—It is always necessary, if possible, to ascertain the cause of the dizziness in order to successfully treat it. If it is due to disease of the heart, absolute quiet is necessary to relieve it; and when it depends on a disordered stomach, that must be attended to. In most cases, whatever may be the exciting cause, the direct one is a fullness of the blood vessels of the brain. This is best relieved by the free use of our Home Liver Pill in doses sufficiently large to have a decided purging effect. In addition to this from ten to fifteen drops of the fluid extract of ergot should be taken three or four times a day, and in severe cases half a teaspoonful may be given at a dose.

SPINAL IRRITATION.

Tenderness along the spine accompanied by an uneasy ache and a feeling of general languor is commonly spoken of as spinal irritation. It is always due to diseases of some of the internal organs, and is more common with women who are suffering from disease of the womb, and with young girls whose menstrual (monthly) periods have not been properly established.

Treatment.—Rest in the recumbent position is often necessary, but in all cases a surgeon should be consulted with the view of ascertaining if some mechanical support is not needed. Women would always be benefited by using our Tonic Pill for Women, and men will find our Nerve Tonic Pill a valuable remedy. In all cases, however, it is necessary to find out what the cause of the spinal irritation is and to remove the same if possible.

CONVULSIONS.

The convulsions so commonly met with in children are all due to some form of direct or reflex irritation of the nervous system. The irritation of teething, the presence of worms, undigested food and inflammation of the stomach and bowels, are the most common causes.

Treatment.—The cause must always be ascertained and properly treated in all cases of convulsions. When a paroxysm is on, or threatened, the feet and hands should be put in hot mustard water and from three to five drops of tincture of gelsemium given in a teaspoonful of water, to a child under five years of age. If the head is hot and the face red, cold applications should be made to the head,

EPILEPSY.

Epilepsy, or '' falling sickness '' as it is sometimes called, is a nervous disease in which a sudden loss of consciousness and convulsions characterize an attack. The attacks come on at longer or shorter intervals, depending on the condition of the patient and the excitement to which he may be exposed.

Headache, dizziness, and confusion of mind, usually precede an attack, and in some cases the patient feels as if a current of cold air was blowing upon him, and extending from the feet upward. The patient falls sudden'y, and the fit is characterized by the paleness of the face, violent convulsions of all the muscles of the body, rigidity of the jaw, the eyes open and staring, and frothing at the mouth. A paroxysm may last from a few seconds to several minutes, after which it will cease for a short time and then recur as before. The patient may be rational in a few minutes after an attack, or may know nothing for several days. In either case he has no knowledge of what had occurred. Weeks or months may pass before another attack; but if the case is not properly treated, the attacks become more frequent and severe till finally a complete loss of mental power occurs.

Treatment —During a convulsion nothing can be done, and any effort to give medicine is useless. After a paroxysm, however, thirty drops of tincture of gelsemium should be given in a little water as

soon as the patient can swallow, and this can be repeated every half hour, if there is a recurrence, till
the paroxysms are entirely controlled.

These cases need long and careful treatment,
and often each case needs something entirely different from any other. We prefer to prescribe for
each case individually as the medicine may have to
be varied according to the symptoms in each case.
Whenever a description of a case is sent to us, we
will send the necessary medicine at the standard
price of one dollar for one hundred pills or tablets.

ST. VITUS DANCE.

St. Vitus Dance, or Chorea, is usually a disease
of childhood though it is sometimes met with in
adults. It is a condition of involuntary and irregular spasmodic movements of muscles, and is properly a sympathetic nervous derangement, caused by
irritation of certain nerves, resulting from indigestion, rheumatism, disturbances of the heart action,
intestinal worms, and general debility from previous
disease.

Treatment.—There are so many conditions that
may produce this disorder that a physician should
always be called to ascertain the cause of the disease. In girls it is often caused by delay in the
appearance of the menses (monthly periods); while
irritation of the head of the penis by a long foreskin often causes it in boys. In the latter case an
operation is the only thing that will relieve it. The

cause of the disturbance must be properly treated and the patient supplied with the most nutritious diet.

HYSTERIA.

Hysteria, or Hysterics, is a peculiar sympathetic derangement of the nervous system, affecting the nerves of motion and sensation, and in severe cases even deranging the mind. It was formerly thought to occur only in women, but more recent investigations show that men also suffer from it. In women it is invariably associated with some disturbance of the womb, while men suffer from it after severe mental prostration following other diseases, especially long-standing disorders of digestion. The symptoms are those of uneasiness, extreme anxiety, and general depression of spirits, although at times the patient seems unusually joyful, laughs inordinately without cause, and the next minute will break down and cry as if suffering some terrible affliction. The limbs are stiff and painful, there are noises in the ears and confusion of mind, a feeling as if a ball or lump was stuck in the throat and cannot be moved, pulling of the hair, grating of the teeth, and sometimes spasms. While an attack lasts the patient is often uncontrollable, will abuse the attendants and friends, and scream, laugh, and cry alternately. During this time the heart's action is very irregular, the breathing difficult, and the face is livid and swollen. Great mental excitement

following a period of depression, the sensation of
the lump in the throat, and the belief that a variety
of diseases is developing, are some of the symptoms
of the milder forms of the disease.   Exertion of all
kinds causes great fatigue, the appetite is lost, and
the patient becomes pale and thin.   It seldom happens that such persons are willing to admit that
anything is the matter with them while the paroxysm is present, while they complain of all kinds of
imaginary diseases as soon as the paroxysm passes
over.   The nervous system gradually becomes so
prostrared that the patient can hardly walk or even
sit up, and some decided treatment is necessary to
effect a speedy change.

Treatment.—In the treatment of this disorder
special attention must be given to the hygienic
conditions.   Moderate exercise in the open air is
desirable, and the food must be of the most nutritious character.   Beef, mutton, animal broths, etc.,
should constitute the diet, while starches and sugar
should be practically avoided.   Tight lacing and
heavy skirts suspended from the hips always aggravate the trouble.   No treatment is complete that
does not see that these things are avoided.   Internally our Tonic Pills for Women should be used
regularly as directed during the day time, and our
Neurodine Tablet should be given every night at
bedtime.   When a hysterical paroxysm is approaching, or after one has occurred, and there are indi-
cations of a re-occurrence, our Neurodine Tablet

should be given every half hour until the nervous excitement is quieted down and the patient feels comfortable. In all cases a careful examination should be made to ascertain the exact cause of the disease, and whenever uterine troubles are recognized these should be specially treated. It is also important that the bowels should be regular. Where the least constipation or coated tongue is present our Home Liver Pills should be used until the bowels move regularly.

HICCOUGH.

Hiccough is a peculiar noise caused by the contractions of the windpipe and muscles of the chest, which is so familiar to every one that it requires no description. It is due to inflammatory conditions of the stomach, bowels, and liver, and is a common symptom of chronic indigestion. When it occurs after a protracted illness of an acute character it is a very unfavorable symptom, as it frequently indicates the near approach of death.

Treatment.—A sudden start or fright will often arrest a paroxysm of hiccough, as will also a dash of cold water in the face, or a drink of cold water. Ten drops of hartshorn in a wine glass of water, taken in one dose, will also frequently counteract it. When it occurs frequently, and especially after eating, our Dyspepsia Pills should be used to correct the disordered digestion and our Home Liver Pills should be taken at bedtime to regulate the bowels.

SEA-SICKNESS.

Considerable attention has been given to the faintness, nausea, and vomiting, from which most people suffer during the first few days at sea, and various remedies have been suggested, but few if any have given the desired relief.

The treatment should be preventive rather than curative, and a person contemplating a sea voyage should always prepare the system by a light diet for a few days, and the free use of our Home Liver Pills every night until the bowels have been freely moved. Twenty grains of bromide of sodium when taken every three hours after going on shipboard is also claimed to have a good effect in preventing sea-sickness. This remedy does certainly agree with many people, and seems to have a soothing influence on the nervous system, and thus prevents the nervous shocks incidental to the motion of the vessel. When the sickness occurs nothing but free vomiting will give any relief. After this occurs the juice of a lemon in about a tablespoonful of water, without sugar, taken several times a day, often overcomes the nausea and faintness. In other cases again a tablespoonful of brandy proves the best remedy; but as no two cases are exactly alike, neither can they be treated in the same way. There is no doubt, however, that when the stomach and liver are in a healthy condition, and care is taken in the diet during the early stages of the voyage, the sea-sickness will be either entirely absent or very slight.

NEURALGIA.

Neuralgia is a disease due to a congestion of the affected nerves. There may be simply a condition of increased sensibility, but usually it extends so as to cause intense pain of the darting, shooting character. The disease may occur in any part of the body, but the face and thigh are the parts most frequently affected.

Neuralgia may be produced by any condition that lowers the vitality of the body, while exposure to cold, malarial influences, and injuries of the nerves themselves, are the most common causes. Sometimes a decayed tooth will expose the nerve of the tooth, and thus give rise not only to toothache but to facial neuralgia. The pain is of the dull, aching character at first, which comes on gradually and is attended by numbness; but it soon becomes sharp, and of the darting, cutting character. At one time it may be confined to some particular part, and again it will run along the course of the nerve both toward the extremity and toward the trunk. The pain is often intense and may be associated with symptoms of fever. It often happens that attacks of neuralgia come on periodically, and in such cases they are invariably associated with malarial conditions, and the skin is usually dry and hot, the tongue is

coated, the appetite poor, and the bowels constipated.

Tic-douloureux, or Facial Neuralgia, is a term
applied to the disease when it spreads over the
entire one side of the face, and in this condition it will also extend so that it would seem
as if all the teeth on that side are affected by the
pain.

Sciatica is a name given to neuralgia affecting
the sciatic nerve, which is a large nerve formed by
the union of several branches of nerves from the
lower part of the spine. It runs down the outer
side of the thigh, behind a portion of the hip joint.
In this form of the disease the pain begins in the
back and runs down through the hip and thigh to
the knee. The suffering in these cases is intense
and may continue for weeks or even months.

Treatment.—In all cases of neuralgia the patient
should be kept as quiet as possible. The bowels
should be regulated by our Home Liver Pills taken
every night until the desired effect is produced.
For the relief of the pain there is no remedy equal
to our Neurodine Tablets, which will invariably
cure the worst cases of neuralgia when used according to directions. This will not only relieve
the pain of the affected nerve, but equalizes the
circulation of the blood in the nerve centers, and
thus removes the principal exciting cause of the
disease. When there are evidences of periodicity
that indicate malarial origin, our Malarial Pills

should be used freely as directed until the periodi-cal attacks disappear.

The same general treatment is necessary for sciatica, but it may also be necessary to apply a mustard plaster or even a fly blister to relieve the severity of the pain. Sometimes stretching the leg will serve a good purpose. In addition to this an electric current will be found of great benefit, espe-cially that obtained from the Earth-Magneto Elec-tric Battery, for the proper use of which see page 262 It must always be borne in mind that sciatica is entirely different from rheumatism, and remedies that are proper especially for the treatment of rheu-matism do not have any effect on sciatica. The name sciatic rheumatism is a misnomer and often leads people to use remedies that can give no pos-sible relief for the symptoms of this disease.

PARALYSIS.

Paralysis is a loss of motion and sensation, either partial or complete, of some part of the body. It is not itself a disease, but is a symptom of various diseases of brain and spinal cord. It will often happen that the primary cause may in a great measure disappear while the paralyzed condition of the extremities may continue for some time after-wards. A paralysis may affect one arm or leg, or both legs, or it may affect one entire side of the body. In some cases paralysis occurs suddenly, while again it develops gradually until either motion or sensation is entirely lost. Sometimes the motion is entirely lost while the sensation is perfect, while in other cases the patient may have perfect motion with an entire loss of sensation. Whatever the cause of paralysis, whenever it once occurs, long treatment is necessary to restore the affected parts to their natural condition.

Treatment.—The conditions giving rise to the paralysis should be ascertained if possible, by a competent physician and treated as the circumstances of the case may require.

In addition to this our Nerve Tonic Pill should be used regularly as long as there is any indication of defective motion or sensation. The bowels should be kept regular by the use of our Home Liver Pills, and attention should be given to providing a nutritious diet. Solids should be avoided as a diet, as much as possible, for the digestion is naturally feeble, and liquid foods of easy digestion should be provided.

CHAPTER VIII.

Disease of the Heart.

PALPITATION OF THE HEART—RHEUMATISM OF THE
HEART—DISEASES OF THE VALVES—ENLARGE-
MENT OF THE HEART—FATTY DEGENERATION
—ANGINA PECTORIS.

The diseases that affect the structure of the heart
are of such a character that they are rarely recognized until they have become well advanced. Few
of them can be successfully diagnosed or treated
without the aid of the experienced physician, and
it would therefore be useless to attempt any description of them in a treatise of this character. The
various valvular diseases of the heart either develop
as a result of some other organic disease, or in their
turn give rise to disease of some other organ; and
the symptoms associated with them are usually
difficult breathing, cough, mucus secretion from the
bronchial tubes, bloody expectoration and hæmor-
rhage. These conditions are usually followed by
dropsy of the abdomen as well as of the feet and
legs. No general line of treatment can be laid
down without knowing the exact nature of the

trouble, and for this purpose the physician must always be consulted.

PALPITATION OF THE HEART.

The heart's action often becomes irregular in consequence of some sympathetic disturbance which is associated with diseases of the stomach, liver, or lungs; and it is so violent that the patient imagines he has some serious organic disease of the heart. This irregular action is usually called palpitation, and is always liable to be recognized by the patient, while organic diseases of the heart escape attention for a considerable length of time.

The usual symptoms of palpitation are a dull pain in the region of the heart, rapid tremulous beating, a sense of choking, difficult breathing, and sometimes a feeling as if the heart was turned over; dizziness, faintness, coldness of the skin, and clammy perspiration are always present. These symptoms are always aggravated by lying on the left side, and are always increased when the stomach is distended with food or accumulated gases. The attacks may come on suddenly after walking, soon after a meal, or following an after-dinner smoke. In fact excessive smoking will invariably give rise to palpitation of the heart, and if it is persisted in for any length of time this functional disturbance will gradually develop some organic change in the structure of the heart itself, thus constituting a genuine heart disease,

Treatment.—Derangements of digestion or general nervous prostration must be relieved in all cases where palpitation of the heart constitutes a prominent symptom. The hygienic condition of the patient must always be seen to, and fresh air, especially during the night, good food, and regular habits, are of the first importance. In all cases of this character the heart disturbance is sympathetic, or functional, as it is sometimes called, and with a view of relieving the immediate attack two of our Neurodine Tablets may be given at a dose and repeated in half an hour, if necessary, to give relief. When constipation is present our Home Liver Pill must be used to overcome it, and the special disease occasioning the palpitation must be treated before permanent relief can be obtained. It can, however, be laid down as a general rule that when a person complains of irregular action of the heart, and is constantly dreading death from heart disease, the disorder is of this character, and not organic.

RHEUMATISM OF THE HEART.

When acute rheumatism attacks different joints and muscles in succession, it is liable to affect the muscular structure of the heart, thus producing rheumatism of the heart. When this condition develops, the severe pain usually leaves the parts of the body that were first attacked.

In mild cases there is a dull pain in the region of the heart, which lasts for a few moments, and then lets up for a short interval. There is also a feeling of great depression, and a difficulty of breathing, as in all heart troubles. The pulsations of the heart are usually strong, and impart a motion to the walls of the chest; while the pulse is quick and irregular, and the extremities become cold. The action of the skin, kidneys, and bowels, become obstructed, and more or less headache is liable to develop.

In severe cases the pain is sharp and boring, and a pronounced chill is felt. The body becomes hot, while the face and extremities are cold and bathed in a clammy perspiration. The pain is felt most with each pulsation, and the patient will usually press his hands to his sides to restrict the motion, and thus obtain relief.

Treatment.—When such symptoms follow an attack of rheumatism a physician should be sent for at once, as such cases are serious, and require immediate attention. Till the doctor arrives relief may be obtained by applying a large mustard plaster over the region of the heart, with the patient in a semi-recumbent position. If at hand, one of our Neurodine Tablets may be given every half hour till four or five doses are taken.

If a person has had one attack of rheumatism of the heart, he is liable to have another; therefore care should be taken to resort to the use of our Rheumatic Pills, when the first twinges of rheumatic pains are felt in any part of the body.

DISEASES OF THE VALVES.

The several valves, or gates of the heart, are liable to be affected, and thus produce irregular action of the heart, which can only be recognized by a careful examination by a physician. Whenever any irregular heart action is felt a physician should be consulted at once, before the serious complications of dropsy and bronchial irritation are developed.

ENLARGEMENT OF THE HEART

The heart may be enlarged by an increase in the muscular structure of the organ or by a dilatation of the cavities. Sometimes both these conditions are present, and the heart can then perform its functions, almost normally for years, without any special inconvenience.

The only thing to be done by a person suffering from this form of heart trouble is to frequently consult a competent physician, to live regularly, and to avoid all violent exercise.

FATTY DEGENERATION OF THE HEART.

By Fatty Degeneration of the Heart is meant a gradual change of the muscular structure of the heart into fatty tissue. This occurs in persons who are disposed to grow fat. The usual symptoms are a small, weak, irregular pulse, slow respiration, and a feeling of faintness on the slightest exertion;

but long before any other symptom is noticed the patient will find a difficulty of breathing on going up stairs, or walking fast.

Treatment.—A nutritious diet, free from starches, sugars, and fats, is of the first importance, and some good nerve tonic is also of great value. In the absence of a physician our Nerve Tonic Pills will do much to increase the strength and improve the general condition of the sufferer.

ANGINA PECTORIS.

Angina Pectoris, or Neuralgia of the Heart, is a disease that begins with an intense, cutting, darting pain in the heart, which soon extends over the entire chest and causes severe muscular contractions. Sometimes it is connected with organic diseases of the heart and arteries, but it often comes on as an independent disease.

It comes on without warning while the patient is following his usual avocation, or even during sleep. The pain extends to the left arm and side of the neck, and causes great agony, and a sense of suffocation. The agony may last but a few minutes, or it may continue for two or three hours. When the disease first shows itself there is usually a long interval between the attacks, but after a time they recur more frequently, and finally may come on at any time.

Treatment.—To relieve the severity of the pain during an attack two of our Neurodine Tablets should be taken every half hour till the pain is relieved, or till three doses are taken. To prevent a recurrence the best known remedy is nitroglycerin, which should be taken in pill form, in doses of one one-hundredths of a grain three times a day.

CHAPTER IX.

Urinary Diseases.

CONGESTION AND INFLAMMATION OF THE KIDNEYS
—BRIGHT'S DISEASE—GRAVEL—RETENTION OF
URINE — INFLAMMATION OF THE BLADDER —
STONE IN THE BLADDER — INVOLUNTARY ES-
CAPE OF URINE.

Under the title of Urinary Diseases are included
the several disorders of the kidneys, the ureter (or
passage leading from the kidneys to the bladder),
the bladder, and the urethra, or outlet of the bladder. The condition of these organs is very important to the general health of the system, as their
function is to remove from the body materials that
are no longer essential to the support of the tissues.
Such ingredients are removed from the blood by
the kidneys and are discharged with the urine.
A healthy adult will pass about thirty-six ounces or
a little over a quart of urine per day. When there
is a perceptible increase or diminution in this quantity, or when the color varies materially from a
clear amber hue, it is wise to ascertain whether any
disturbance of these organs exists, as the success of
treatment depends upon beginning in their early

stages, before any material change of structure has taken place.

CONGESTION AND INFLAMMATION OF THE KIDNEYS.

As a result of exposure to cold the kidneys may become congested, and this congestion may extend to acute inflammation of the part. This condition occasions pain in the region of the kidneys, extending downward toward the bladder, and a frequent desire to pass water. Only a small quantity of water is voided at each effort, and after a time some blood is mixed with the urine. The skin is dry and hot, nausea is sometimes present, and the patient is irritable and restless. The urine for a time becomes scanty, and delirium and stupor set in, as the result of the poisoning of the blood by the retention of the effete material that should be thrown off.

Treatment.—The object of the treatment is to relieve the kidneys as much as possible. This is best done by procuring a free perspiration and copious action of the bowels. The patient should be kept quiet, hot fomentations or poultices should be applied over the kidneys, and ten grains of Dover's Powder will often be found of great service in quieting the pain and promoting the perspiration. H o m e Liver Pills should be used to promote a free action of the bowels, and as soon as the acute symptoms subside remedies should be used to promote the action of the kidneys. For this purpose our

H o m e Kidney Pill should be given every three
or four hours until the urine flows freely. Absolute
quiet on the part of the patient is essential to a
speedy reduction of the inflammatory condition.

Bright's disease is the name usually given to
that form of derangement of the kidneys where a
change in the structure of the kidneys has followed
an acute or chronic inflammation of that organ. It
is characterized by the presence of a white substance in the urine which is called albumen, and
this can always be detected in the urine by the thick
sediment which forms after boiling the urine or
adding a small quantity of nitric acid to it.

The first symptoms of this disease are a general
condition of weakness, scanty urine, and deposit of
a white sediment in the urine after standing, dropsical swelling of the feet and legs, and the presence
in the urine of albumen. This can only be recognized by a chemical and microscopical examination
of the urine, and this should be made with great
care, because many physicians make grave mis-
takes in diagnosis from not properly understanding
how to examine the urine chemically or failing to
examine it under the microscope. Any person sus-
pecting the presence of Bright's disease should at
the earliest possible time have the urine examined
by some one competent to do so, and if the slightest
trace of albumen is present, though it may not nec-

essarily indicate the presence of Bright's disease, it should at least warn the patient of possible danger ahead, and immediate treatment should be begun with a view of preventing any possible change of the structure of the kidneys, or any development of the disease.

Treatment.—Much has been said about the treatment of Bright's disease, and many remedies have been offered to the public as specifics that were sure to cure it. Many of these remedies have been valuable and have deservedly obtained fame as curatives for Bright's disease. It is unfortunate, however, that it is claimed for such remedies that they are capable of curing all the evils flesh is heir to. It should be borne in mind, and the sooner the lesson is learned the better, that medicines that will relieve the uncomfortable symptoms of Bright's disease cannot by any possibility have any effect upon the other organs and structures of the body. The object to be attained in the treatment of Bright's disease is to arrest the destruction of the tissue of the kidneys, and to do this remedies are necessary that will produce excessive secretion of the urine. When taken in time, and persistently followed according to directions, we believe our Home Kidney Pills will be found to promptly relieve those conditions of the kidneys where albumen is present in the urine before there is much breaking down of the structure of the kidneys. This pill should therefore be taken with the first appearance of the disease, and continued for months, with a view of relieving the kidneys of unnecessary work, and thereby preventing the further development of Bright's disease. We do not say that all cases can be cured, for it is a well-known fact that when the structure of the kidneys has entirely changed no amount of treatment can restore it, and consequently the disease cannot be arrested; but in many cases it may stop before it extends to the destruction of the kidney itself, and in such cases the H o m e Kidney Pills will be found the best remedy that can be employed. It is necessary, however, that the disease should be properly diagnosed before any medicine is used.

With a view of affording our readers the advantage of a careful chemical and microscopical examination of the urine, for proper diagnosis of this and other diseases of the kidneys and bladder, we agree, on receiving a sample of urine, with three dollars, to return a complete analysis and diagnosis of the case. This examination would cost ten dollars to any person consulting any of our physicians in their private offices.

GRAVEL.

Gravel is an accumulation of earthy materials in the form of minute concretions, resembling gravel stones, which develop in the kidneys and pass from them to the bladder through the passage which conveys the urine. The passage of these little stones through this narrow canal occasions in most instances intense pain, which is of a sharp, deep-seated, cutting character. It begins in the region of one kidney and passes downward along the groin toward the bladder, changing location as the gravel stones advance, and finally it ceases on the escape of the gravel stones into the bladder. During the passage of these stones there is a frequent desire to urinate, attended by a scalding pain, but only a few drops of urine can be voided at a time. The passage of the stone may take place in an hour or so, or may occupy several days, during which time the patient suffers intensely. After the gravel has passed into the bladder, it may sometimes be seen or felt escaping through the urethra; and persons who are once attacked by this disease are liable to be so again, and after a time he may even suffer from stone in the bladder.

Treatment.—As nothing is known of the nature of the trouble until the stone begins to pass from the kidneys, preventive treatment is at first unthought of. During the attack the only thing that can be done is to ease the pain and relax the tension of the canal through which the stone is passing. This is best accomplished by the use of our Neurodine Tablets, of which two should be taken at a dose, and in severe cases two more after an interval of half an hour. They can be repeated three or four times if the pain is not relieved. With a view of preventing a recurrence of the trouble, one of

HomeKidney Pill should be taken four or five times a day for several weeks. It is an absolute cure for gravel, even in its worst form, if taken according to the directions.

When a brick-dust sediment is seen in the urine, fifteen drops of nitro-muriatic acid in half a gobletful of water should be taken three or four times a day. The entire quantity should be taken at once through a glass tube, and it is very essential to dilute it thus largely so as to prevent undue irritation of the stomach.

RETENTION OF URINE.

Sometimes a full quantity of urine may be excreted by the kidneys, and yet it will accumulate in the bladder, without the ability to pass it. This is sometimes caused by an effort to retain the urine for a long time after the desire to void it occurs. If may also be due to a paralysis of the bladder or a contraction of the neck of the bladder, resulting from cold or the presence of piles. When the urine is retained there is a sense of fullness associated with pain in the lower part of the abdomen, and after a time the pain and pressure with the desire to urinate becomes very severe, while every effort to void the urine only seems to make matters worse.

Treatment.—Hot cloths, or a hot fomentation of hops, applied over the region of the bladder will often start the urine. Sitting in a tub of hot water so that the water comes over the abdomen, up to the navel, will also serve the same purpose. If this fails to relieve the patient, the physician should be sent for and the water drawn off with a catheter. In many cases there may be stricture, or some form of mechanical obstruction which gives rise to this condition, and when such is the case proper surgical treatment should be sought.

INFLAMMATION OF THE BLADDER.

The lining membrane of the bladder may be affected by acute or chronic inflammation which may result from cold or external injuries, the continued and excessive use of medicines that are intended to increase the flow of urine, the pressure of a displaced womb on the bladder, and inflammation extending from neighboring parts to the bladder itself. The symptoms are a dull pain in the lower part of the abdomen, frequent desire to pass water, with increased pain with every effort to do so, scanty and high colored urine, scalding sensation along the entire course of the canal, a feeling of contraction or spasm at the neck of the bladder, and sometimes a chill, followed by fever, which may continue for several days.

These symptoms are not quite so severe in chronic inflammation of the bladder, but are of the same general character. A thick white sediment is present in the urine, and sometimes it sticks to the vessel in the form of a slimy mass. The smell is putrid and the urine is entirely void of acid. The bowels are usually constipated, the appetite poor, the skin dry and sallow, and when long continued there is a failure of strength and flesh.

Treatment.—The hot hip-bath and hot hop fomentations, are valuable in any stage of the disease. Our Neurodine Tablet may be used to relieve spasm and irritation of the neck of the bladder, and our H o m e Kidney Pill will be valuable in increasing the flow of urine, allaying the irritation and relieving the pain. In chronic inflammation it is often necessary to have the bladder washed out by the introduction of a soft rubber catheter, through which a solution of warm water and golden seal is injected into the bladder. In fact, the only radical cure of chronic inflammation of the bladder is secured by placing the patient in bed and persistently following this treatment for three or four months. Without washing out the bladder and absolute rest no cure can be effected, and it is therefore always advisable for persons afflicted with this form of chronic bladder disease to seek treatment at some health resort or sanitarium where such cases can receive the proper attention.

STONE IN THE BLADDER.

Stone in the bladder can only be recognized after a careful examination on the part of the surgeon, but the general symptoms invariably point to the nature of the trouble. With stone in the bladder the sense of irritation and burning is always felt when the bladder is emptied, while in inflammation of the bladder these sensations are present when the bladder is full.   While voiding the urine the stream will start freely and full, but be suddenly stopped before the act is complete. After a moment's delay it may begin again and be again stopped, and this is repeated two or three times before the water is entirely voided.   These symptoms alone conclusively point to the presence of stone in the bladder, but it should be confirmed by the examination of the surgeon.

An operation is the only means by which this trouble can be relieved, and it should not be delayed after the case is properly diagnosed.

INVOLUNTARY ESCAPE OF URINE.

The involuntary escape of urine from the b'adder is called incontinence of urine.   It occurs as a consequence of paralysis of the neck of the bladder, or some form of irritation which causes the bladder to contract after a small quantity of urine is accumulated in it.   It is a condition that is frequently met with in young children and after protracted sickness.   When it takes place it is very distressing, as it soils the clothing and produces excoriation of the skin of the adjacent parts.

Treatment.—In cases where the condition is due to a tendency to muscular contraction of the neck of the bladder, the following mixture will certainly effect a cure: Tincture of belladonna, thirty drops; water, eight tablespoonfuls. Mix, and give a teaspoonful every two or three hours. If the trouble is due to a relaxed condition of the neck of the bladder, from one to two drops of the tincture of nux vomica should be given in a little water two or three times a day.

If one of these remedies is tried, and should fail to produce the desired effect after a couple of weeks' trial, the other should be resorted to for the same length of time, and if both of them fail, it is best that a physician should be consulted.

CHAPTER X.

Special Diseases of Men.

GONORRHEA, OR CLAP — GLEET—BALANITIS — PHY-
MOSIS— PARAPHIMOSIS— STRICTURE—SWELLED
TESTICLES— HYDROCELE—VARICOCELE— SELF-
ABUSE—SPERMATORRHEA.

The generative organs of men are affected by a variety of diseases, some of which are developed from ordinary causes, while others result from specific poisons transmitted through impure coitus. These diseases are usually spoken of as " Venereal Diseases," or " Private Diseases," and in consequence of their nature more humbug has been praeticed in connection with their treatment than in any other department of medicine.

Sufferers should shun such public advertisers as announce " No cure, no pay," " The oldest specialist," " Twenty-five years' experience," etc., etc., as they are invariably men of no experience, who aim to profit by the credulity of their unfortunate victims.

These diseases are as amenable to successful treatment as any others, and when once properly cured leave the patient as free from subsequent disorders as though they had never occurred.

As a result of impure sexual intercourse a local sore on the genitals often results, which is known as a chancre, or pox, and from this is developed a constitutional blood disease which has already been treated of on page 76.

Of the other diseases of the genitals, the most common are gonorrhea and its complications which result from impure sexual intercourse, and a number of functional disorders, and anatomical and physiological abnormalities.

GONORRHEA, OR CLAP.

Gonorrhea, or clap, is a specific disease resulting from impure coitus. In the male it affects the urethra, or urinary passage, and causes an inflammation which is accompanied by a profuse discharge.

An uneasy tickling sensation is felt in the head of the penis in from two to five days after exposure. A clear whitish discharge then appears, which soon becomes thick and yellow. A severe smarting or burning sensation is felt each time the urine is passed, while the head of the penis and the foreskin becomes swollen and red. Sometimes there is a general condition of fever which lasts for several days, and after three or four days the patient often experiences painful erections during the night.

Treatment.—As soon as any of these symptoms are recognized, and especially when a discharge from the penis is seen a few days after promiscuous intercourse, a proper treatment should be adopted to insure a speedy cure of the disease.

With the view of insuring secrecy and an absolute certainty of a speedy cure, we have prepared a tablet which is readily dissolved in water, and also a capsule to take internally, which will cure such cases in a few days. One of our H o m e Specific Tablets, three times a day, used as directed, in connection with our H o m e Specific Pills, will cure this disease more promptly and certainly than any other known treatment.

GLEET.

Gleet is simply a chronic form of gonorrhea, and is never met with except as a result of badly treated cases of " clap." There is no pain, heat, or swelling in this condition, but there is a slight discharge of a clear, viscid fluid, which sticks the lips of the meatus together. In some cases the stream of water is considerably smaller than normal.

Treatment.—In these cases a radical cure can be effected by the use of our H o m e Specific Tablet No. 2 as directed. You can treat yourself at home with the certainty of having an absolute cure.

If this treatment does not give satisfactory results, we may have reason to suspect the presence of a stricture, when an experienced surgeon should be consulted, and measures adopted at once to overcome the stricture.

BALANITIS.

Balanitis is an inflammation of the mucous membrane lining the foreskin and covering the head of the penis. It may be caused by irritation from any cause, lack of cleanliness, or the contact of the gonorrheal poison. The parts become very tender and much swollen, and often a free discharge is thrown off from the surface.

Treatment.—Draw back the foreskin and thoroughly cleans the parts with warm water. Then dissolve one of our H o m e Specific Tablets in two tablespoonfuls of water, and bathe the parts thoroughly two or three times a day.

PHYMOSIS.

When the foreskin is drawn over the head of the penis and so constricted that it cannot be pushed back, the condition is called Phymosis. This results in an annoying inflammation of the head of the penis and the foreskin, which can only be relieved by a proper surgical operation.

If you hesitate to consult your family physician, we can direct you where to go to have the operation successfully performed. When necessary such an operation should not be delayed a moment, as the normal conditions of the parts are restored as soon as the operation is properly performed.

Sometimes the foreskin is unnaturally long from birth, and this gives rise to frequent attacks of inflammation. In all such cases the operation known as circumcision should be performed as early as possible, for an elongated foreskin usually prevents the normal development of the penis.

PARAPHIMOSIS.

Paraphimosis is a condition in which the foreskin is drawn back behind the head of the penis, and becomes so inflamed that it cannot be drawn forward. It seldom occurs except as a complication of gonorrhea or chancre. If it is not promptly relieved it so constricts the head of the penis as to cause serious trouble.

If the patient cannot draw down the foreskin by pulling on it with the index and second fingers and pushing up the head with the thumbs, a physician should be consulted at once.

STRICTURE.

A stricture is a contraction of the urinary passage that prevents the free passage of the urine from the bladder. It is caused by gonorrhea or a chancre in the canal, or by some direct local injury.

The more common symptoms are frequent desire to urinate, a gleety discharge, a decrease in the size of the stream of urine, or a dividing or twisting of the stream, If neglected the canal gradually closes till finally it is almost impossible to void the urine.

These cases cannot be treated at home, and the most approved methods do away entirely with cutting, which was formerly attended by such serious results. Those applying to us will be advised how and where to get the best scientific treatment.

SWELLED TESTICLE.

An enlarged condition of the testicle frequently results from inflammation of the organ following gonorrhea or direct local injury.

On the start the pain is severe and the swelling increases the size of the organ to three or four times its normal condition. Such cases require the immediate attention of a skilled surgeon.

When the enlargement becomes chronic a specialist should be consulted.

HYDROCELE.

Hydrocele is an accumulation of water in the scrotum, or bag. It comes on gradually and often attains enormous size. At first it is not attended with pain or inconvenience, but after a time it becomes an ugly deformity and interferes with or completely destroys the sexual function.

The usual method of treatment is to draw off the water by tapping. When this is done it rapidly fills again, and is soon worse than before.

It is best to consult a reliable specialist from the

start, and have an operation performed for its radical cure.

Our surgeons have had most wonderful success in operating on such cases, and will gladly give an opinion to any of our readers who send us a description of their case.

VARICOCELE.

Varicocele is a diseased condition of the veins of the testicles, which causes them to enlarge and fill the scrotum, and after a time to completely destroy the structure of the testicle.

It is one of the most common causes of spermatorrhea, or loss of manhood, and can only be cured by a radical operation. The sooner an operation is performed in such cases the better the result.

SELF-ABUSE.

By Masturbation, or Self-abuse, is meant the excitation of the sexual organs by mechanical irritation. It is a habit to which both sexes are liable, but boys are more addicted to it than girls. It is also spoken of as self-polution, the secret vice, onanism, etc. It is a vice acquired about the age of puberty, and if persisted in for any length of time it deranges the nervous system, arrests the growth of the body and prevents the normal development of the genital organs.

Parents cannot be too careful in cautioning their children against the terrible evils that are sure to follow this habit.   Boys often learn the evils of this practice too late to prevent the sequences that are sure to follow.   Among these may be mentioned nervous prostration, melancholia, loss of memory, lascivious dreams, nocturnal emissions, and the esc pe of semen in other ways.   This unnatural escape of semen is spoken of as spermatorrhea, which will be next described.

Any young man who is addicted to this vice should have moral strength enough to stop it, and at once, and thus save himself much suffering He will however be greatly aided in his effort by the use of our Home Nerve Tonic Pills, which are so com- blned as to constitute an infallible specific in all such cases, if taken according to the directions.

SPERMATORRHEA.

Spermatorrhea is an escape of seamen without sexual intercourse.   It may occur during the night as the result of a lascivious dream, or it may escape with each passage of the urine.   In persons who have abused the sexual organs in any way the sight of a woman will often produce a seminal discharge.

It is usually present in early manhood, and may be caused by self-abuse, excessive sexual indulg- ence, varicocele, hydrocele, or any wasting nervous disease, or long protracted illness.

If a man has emissions three or four times a month, or oftener, it shows an abnormal weakness of his genital organs, which should be corrected at once, so as to prevent a destruction of manhood.

In all such cases, where the special treatment of an experienced specialist cannot be obtained, our Home Nerve Tonic Pills will give the most satisfactory results, and in many cases will effect a radical cure.

In cases of varicocele or hydrocele an operation for the radical cure of these conditions is essential to a cure of the spermatorrhea.

Persons suffering from this weakness should send to us for our " Question Blanks for Men." By returning the same, with the answers to the questions filled in, we will send them, free of charge, a letter of advice, giving full directions as to the best treatment to be adopted for each individual case.

IMPOTENCE.

Impotence, or loss of manhood, means an inability to perform the marital act. This condition results from self-abuse, excessive sexual indulgence, severe mental strain, worry, protracted sickness, and impaired nutrition. It may occur at any period of life, but is most commonly met with in young men who have practiced self-abuse, and in those who have indulged in sexual excesses.

Home Nerve Tonic Pills will prove the most valuable remedy that can be used at home for all recent cases; but in all long standing cases the proper application of electricity, and special treatment for each case can be prescribed, so as to insure a radical cure.

We will give advice, free of charge, to all persons who send for and answer our "Question Blank for Men;" and from our past experience we can promise a cure in ninty-five per cent. of all cases of impotence.

CHAPTER XI.

Diseases and Injuries of the Skin.

ACNE, OR FLESH WORMS—BED SORES—BOILS—CAR-
BUNCLES— CORNS— CHILBLAINS — DANDRUFF—
FALLING OUT OF THE HAIR—ECZEMA—FRECK-
LES—NETTLE RASH, OR HIVES—PRICKLEY HEAT
—RING WORM—SALT RHEUM—WARTS—ITCH
—BARBERS ITCH—BURNS AND SCALDS.

The skin is liable to be affected by certain diseases, as well as to receive injuries which require
special attention. The most common diseases of
the skin are acne or flesh worms, bed sores, boils,
carbuncles, corns, chilblains, itch, barbers itch,
eczema, dandruff, freckles, moles, nettle rash or
hives, prickly heat, ring worm, scald head, salt
rheum, warts, and falling out of the hair, while
burns and scalds, sunburn and wounds, are the
most common form of accidents.

ACNE, OR FLESH WORMS.

Flesh Worms, as they are commonly called, are
caused by an accumulation of a natural excretion of
the skin remaining in the pores, and the surface
becoming blackened from the dust of the air.

This accumulation, after obstructing the pores of the skin for a time, often acts as a foreign body, thus causing a pimple in which matter forms. After the matter is thus formed, the hardened mass is loosened and can be easily removed. This condition is more commonly present in young persons, especially after the age of puberty, and is invariably due to disordered digestion. The tongue will be found coated, the bowels usually constipated, and the stomach deranged.

Treatment.—The bowels should always be regulated by the use of our H o m e Liver Pill, and where the digestion is deranged our H o m e Dyspepsia Pills should be used as directed. The pores of the skin throughout the body should be kept free and open by frequent bathing, and Turkish or hot baths will invariably be found of great value. The face and shoulders, where these black heads are most commonly noticed, should be bathed at night with hot water and the skin rubbed freely with a coarse wash-cloth, after which the following lotion should be applied:

Nitrate of potash, one ounce; boracic acid, twenty grains; rose water, six ounces. Bathe the face freely with this mixture, and allow it to dry on the skin without wiping.

BED SORES.

Bed sores are ulcerated surfaces of the skin caused by long continued pressure at one point in

persons who are confined to bed during a long illness. To relieve these the pressure should be removed from the affected part by cushions or rubber rings inflated with air, the part should be bathed with warm water and some fine toilet soap, and
if the surface is unhealthy it should be sprinkled
with powdered burnt alum. This should remain
on for a few hours, when it can be washed off and
the part dressed with our H o m e Ointment,
applied on a piece of lint or old linen, two or three
times a day. The surface should be washed each
time the fresh ointment is applied.

BOILS.

A boil is an inflammation of a circumscribed
portion of the skin with the tissue underneath it,
and is usually the result of impure blood, and some
local obstruction of the pores of the skin. Usually
when one boil develops it is succeeded by a number
of others following at regular intervals. The digestion is always impaired, and the organs that carry
off the effete material from the system , are in
some way obstructed when such a condition is
present.

Treatment.—The best method of treating a boil is
to have it lanced deeply upon the first appearance
of the inflammation. This allows the blood to escape freely and the matter will not form.

If this is not done, it should be poulticed with a
hot flax seed meal poultice until it comes to a head.

It should then be opened or squeezed until the matter escapes, after which it should be thoroughly cleansed and dressed with the H o m e Ointment at least twice a day. Attention should be given to the digestive organs, the bowels should be properly regulated, Turkish baths or ordinary hot-water baths should be frequently resorted to, and where more than one occurs our H o m e Alterative Pills should be taken to purify the blood.

CARBUNCLES.

A carbuncle is nothing more or less than a large boil. It may occur on any part of the body but is most commonly met with on the back of the neck. The inflammation often involves the deeper tissues, and in this locality may extend to the roots of the nerves, in which case it may prove fatal. When the surface involved in an inflammation of this kind is extensive and the part tense and hard, an early incision should be made in the inflamed part, and hot poultices should be afterward applied so as to prevent the inflammatory action from extending to the deeper tissues. Usually a hard mass called the core will be thrown off, after which, if the part is thoroughly cleansed, the healing will take place kindly.

CORNS.

Corns are nothing more than thickened cuticle resulting from pressure or friction. They are located usually on the toes, or the joints of the great and little toes, and sometimes on the soles of the feet. Soft corns are situated between the toes. The best method of treating a corn is to soak the feet thoroughly in water as hot as can be borne, and then apply over the surface of the corn our Home Corn Cure, which should be applied on going to bed. It should also be applied for five or six nights in succession, after which the feet should again be soaked in hot water, when the hard cuticle or corn can be very readily peeled off. If this is repeated, and tight shoes are avoided, corns can invariably be radically cured.

CHILBLAINS.

Chilblain is a condition of congestion which usually attacks the skin of the sides of the feet, heels, nose, ears, and fingers, as a result of exposure to cold. It causes a tingling sensation with intense itching, which is likely to continue as long as the cold weather lasts. In some cases the skin becomes ulcerated, and annoying sores are thus produced. The real cause of the trouble is unknown, but it is supposed to be due to an impoverished condition of the blood. The application of snow or cold water to the part will give temporary relief, while the most satisfactory results in the way of treatment are procured by bathing the parts in a

solution of forty drops of carbolic acid to twelve
tablespoonfuls of water.

DANDRUFF.

Dandruff is a disease of the scalp in which there
is redness of the skin and an accumulation of minute scales of a white, dry character. To relieve
the condition, the scalp should be thoroughly washed with a strong solution of powdered borax (one
ounce to the pint of water), after which the head
should be cleansed with clear tepid water. A little
dilute alcohol should then be rubbed into the scalp
every night at bed time for a week or two, and thus
the hair follicles will be so stimulated that the dandruff will be hardly likely to return. A little vaseline or other simple hair dressing can be used in
the morning.

FALLING OUT OF THE HAIR.

The hair is liable to fall out from various causes,
and it has long been the aim of baldheaded people
to find some remedy that would restore the hair to
the bare scalp. Kerosene oil applied every night
has been recommended as a valuable remedy, but
it must be continued for a long time to secure a
good result. Anything by which a thorough friction
of the scalp can be secured will always prove beneficial, so long as there is the slightest evidence of
the roots of the hair being alive. As a simple
dressing, the following will be found serviceable:

Quinine, twelve grains: tannic acid, ten grains; borax, twenty grains; dilute sulphuric acid, ten drops; tincture of Spanish fly, one drachm; glycerine, one ounce; water, five ounces. Mix and use as a hair dressing once a day. It is important, however, that it should be well rubbed into the scalp, and the rubbing continued for five or ten minutes. When the hair is thin, a soft brush should be used to brush the hair thoroughly for fifteen or twenty minutes night and morning.

ECZEMA.

The term Eczema is applied to a great variety of skin eruptions which present themselves in the form of little blisters, secreting a sticky fluid that accumulates on the skin and forms a crust or scab. Pimples of various kinds in which pus forms, and a simple roughness of the skin, are also spoken of as eczema. All troubles of this kind are due to obstruction of the pores of the skin, and to poor blood from defective nutrition. The treatment of eczema must, therefore, be directed to the general hygienic conditions of the patient. Frequent bathing, nutritious diet, and perfect digestion, are essential to a cure of the disease, and such remedies as will relieve any of these defects must be resorted to. In obstinate cases our H o m e Alterative Pill will be found a never-failing remedy for the removal of all blemishes of the skin of the character just described, and our Home Ointment should be applied.

FRECKLES.

The small brown spots on the face and hands of persons of fair complexion which are produced by exposure to the rays of the sun during warm weather are commonly called freckles. These spots are permanently present for a considerable time on young persons, but are always more pronounced during the summer season. They are of slight consequence to most persons, but young ladies are often greatly worried by them. They will, however, find in Kosmema a harmless and pleasant cosmetic that can be used, without showing on the skin, so as to hide the freckles entirely, and after using it for awhile the freckles will be removed.

NETTLE RASH, OR HIVES.

Hives is a disease of childhood which makes its appearance in the form of elevated blotches, attended with heat and intense itching. They are usually white and scattered over different portions of the body. They are due to impaired digestion, and seldom occur excepting as a symptom of impaired digestion and with constipated bowels. They are best treated by an alcohol sweat, or Turkish bath if possible, after which the skin may be bathed with a strong solution of salt and water. The bowels must be regulated by our H o m e Liver Pills, and proper attention should be given to the diet. The heat and itching will be relieved by the H o m e Ointment.

PRICKLEY HEAT.

Prickley Heat is characterized by an eruption of minute bright red spots which thickly cover the skin, as a result of continued over-heating of the body during the extreme hot weather of summer. It is attended by intense itching of a prickling character. A hot bath, or preferably a Turkish bath, will give prompt relief, and the irritation is greatly allayed by the use of our Home Ointment applied freely to the surfaces covered by the rash. This should be applied over the entire surface affected, and renewed night and morning after bathing.

RING WORM.

Ring Worm is a disease of the skin, of a contagious character, caused by the presence of a minute parasite or worm. It shows itself in circular patches, the circumference of which increases in size with the edges elevated and reddened, while the skin in the center retains its natural color. When it attacks the scalp the roots of the hair are destroyed, and the part becomes bald. The best treatment is to apply every night and morning, with a camels-hair brush, pure tincture of iodine. This should be continued until the skin peels off, when it will be found that the parasite has been destroyed. Then the H o m e Ointment should be applied night and morning till a new skin is formed.

SALT RHEUM.

Salt Rheum is a peculiar skin eruption, analogous to eczema, which is characterized by symptoms of general languor, constipation, loss of appetite, and a burning sensation in parts of the skin. Red spots then show themselves at the points and blisters form which contain a clear fluid that soon becomes milky. After four or five days the eruption dries and a scale forms which drops off in a few days leaving a red discoloration of the skin. In the chronic form of the disease the patches become deeply cracked, especially during the cold weather. The acute eruption is usually spoken of as tetter, while the term salt rheum is applied to the chronic form of the disease. The irritation of the skin is promptly relieved and the condition rapidly cured by the application of our H o m e Ointment night and morning. Cleanliness must be rigidly enforced, and fresh air and good diet are essential. An alcohol sweat or Turkish bath will be found serviceable, and the bath should be kept up regularly. In the chronic form of the disease our Home Ointment, night and morning, hould be applied two or three times a day, .vhile internally our H o m e Alterative Pills should be freely administered and continued until all the symptoms of the disease have dis, appeared,

WARTS.

Warts are developed by an enlargement of the minute vascular structure of the skin. They are usually met with in young persons, and may occur singly or in great numbers. They sometimes attain large size but are often small and hard. The old idea that they are contagious and could be communicated by a drop of blood from the wart to the hand of another person is erroneous. An application of chromic acid to the wart will harden the surface so that it can be scraped off the following day. The same application can be made for a number of days in succession, while the hardened tissue is daily removed, and within a week or ten days even long-standing warts can be entirely removed.

ITCH.

The term Itch is applied to a disease of a contagious character, due to the presence of an animal parasite which usually manifests itself between the fingers, and may continue for a long period of time. The best treatment is the application on a pine stick of a little pure carbolic acid directly to the affected part, care being taken not to allow the acid to spread over the healthy skin. This strong application destroys the parasite and the part can then be readily healed by the application of our H o m e Ointment. This ointment should be applied two or three times a day, and a cure is usually effected in eight or ten days.

BARBERS ITCH.

Barbers Itch is another form of skin disease due to the presence of a parasite and is so called because it is often communicated by barbers while shaving their customers. When once developed it may last for months and may often destroy the hair follicles of the mustache and beard. It manifests itself in the form of hard lumps, which often spread over the surface of the cheeks, chin, and upper lip. The same general treatment as that just recommended for itch will be found serviceable in these cases.

BURNS AND SCALDS.

Burns and scalds are conditions in which the skin is wholly or partially destroyed by the application of dry or moist heat. Where the skin is reddeued and the pain of an intense burning character, two heaping teaspoonfuls of baking soda should be put in a teacupful of water, the part should be bathed in this solution and a piece of muslin saturated in the solution should be bound on to the burned part. In a few minutes, the heat and pain will be very much relieved, if not entirely cured. When cases are more severe the main object is to exclude the air until nature can restore the part to its normal condition. This is best douc'hy saturating a piece of lint in a mixture of ten drops of carbolic acid to two tablespoonfuls of sweet oil. The carbolic acid has a soothing, healing effect on the burn, while the oil with the lint excludes the air. In most cases, it is best to leave the lint on until new skin has formed, and the dressing can be renewed by simply pouring carbolized oil over the surface of the lint Sometimes it may be necessary to remove the lint, when the part should be carefully washed with a solution of twenty drops of carbolic acid to a gobletful of water.

COMPOUND TALCUM POWDER.

The original Compound Talcum Powder was introduced to the notice of the profession over twenty years ago by Julius Fehr, M. D. It is a valuable antiseptic and disinfecting powder, which gives good results in the local treatment of all skin diseases. It is also the best powder for general toilet purposes, in caring for infants, and to prevent chafing and all irritation of the skin in adults.

CHAPTER XII.

Diseases of Women.

ABSENCE OF MENSTRUATION—SUPPRESSED MENSTRU-
ATION — PAINFUL MENSTRUATION — PROFUSE
MENSTRUATION—THE VULVA— INFLAMMATION
OF THE VAGINA—INFLAMMATION OF THE WOMB
—ULCERATION OF THE WOMB—LACERATION OF
THE NECK OF THE WOMB—LEUCORRHEA—DIS-
PLACEMENTS OF THE WOMB—LACERATION OF
THE PERINEUM—HYSTERIA—ABSENCE OF CON-
JUGAL DESIRE—STERILITY—TUMORS- CANCERS.

Diseases pecular to women have become so common that they may be said to belong to our modern
civilization. Unnatural modes of dress, such as
tight lacing and high-healed boots, and the violation of the laws of health, are the usual predisposing causes, but there are many exciting causes
which give rise to special forms of these diseases
that may often be avoided.

The functional disorders of women that are usually met with are suppressed menstruation, painful
menstruation, and profuse menstruation.

Menstruation is the general term given to the
monthly flow of blood from the womb, which ac-

companies the discharge of the ovum, or egg, from the ovary. It is popularly spoken of as monthlies, turns, periods, flowers, courses, and being unwell. A healthy girl begins to menstruate at the age of thirteen or fourteen, and the flow is indicative of a normal development of the sexual organs. It should come on without pain or suffering of any kind every twenty-eight days, and should continue for four or five days. Any variation from this rule indicates a departure from health, that should be corrected by proper treatment.

ABSENCE OF MENSTRUATION.

It often happens that girls do not menstruate on arriving at the age of puberty. If they remain undeveloped and have no symptoms of general disturbance of the system it simply indicates a lack of normal development, and no anxiety need be felt till a development of the breasts takes place.

If, however, the girl is fully developed at the age of fourteen, and she suffers from fullness of the head, headaches, flashes of heat in the head and face, and pains in the abdomen, it indicates an effort of nature to establish the menstrual flow. Under such circumstances, if the flow fails to appear an attempt should be made to establish it. In some cases it may be due to a mechanical obstruction of the neek of the womb which will require a surgical operation to relieve; but in the majority of cases there is a congestion of the womb which can be relieved by appropriate remedies. Our H o m e Tonic Pills for Women, if taken according to directions, will relieve the congestion and establish the menstrual flow. Even after the flow has come on the pills should be taken continuously for two or three months, so as to insure the regular recurrence of the periods.

PAINFUL MENSTRUATION.

Many girls and women suffer severe pain just before or during the menstrual periods. When the pain occurs before the flow begins, it indicates a congested or engorged condition of the neck of the womb, which narrows the canal through which the blood passes. When the blood begins to escape the congestion is relieved and the pain is diminished or entirely disappears.

When the pain continues during the entire period, it usually indicates a constriction of the neck of the womb, which is permanent in character.

Treatment.—In all cases of painful menstruation our H o m e Tonic Pills for Women should be used continuously during the month between the periods, and if continued for two or three months they will positively relieve all cases of painful menstruation due to a congested condition of the womb. When these pills fail to give absolute relief, it will be a sure indication that the pain is caused by a constriction or narrowness of the neck of the womb.

In such cases a radical cure can be effected by a

proper dilatation of the neck of the womb. By our modern methods this can be done without cutting, and a radical cure can be guaranteed in every case.

When this trouble is neglected, serious diseases of the womb are sure to develop, sooner or later, and in all cases sterility or barrenness is sure to result.

PROFUSE MENSTRUATION.

Profuse menstruation means an excessive flow of blood during each menstrual period. It may occur as a result of general weakness from some previous disease, after abortions, and when a woman gets up too soon after childbirth. It always exhausts the patient, and in many cases confines them to the bed for several days each month.

Treatment.—During the flow, quiet in the recumbent position is necessary. In the interval between the periods, our H o m e Tonic Pills for Women should be taken and continued for two or three months. In the majority of cases these pills will effect a radical cure. When they fail, however, a specialist should be consulted, as an operation for scraping the inside of the womb, or removing some foreign growth may be required.

THE VULVA.

The Vulva is the general name given to the female external organs of generation. These are the greater and lesser lips, the clitoris, and the hymen.

These parts are liable to inflammation from various causes, when they become hot, painful, and swollen. An itching burning sensation is also present, and there may be a discharge from the parts.

Hot applications should be made to the parts, and the surface bathed freely with the following: fluid hydrastis, one ounce; laudanum, one ounce; water, one pint. Mix, and apply freely every two hours. The patient should remain quiet in bed during the continuance of the inflammation. Sometimes small tumors or lumps will develop on the sides of the vulva, and as soon as they are discovered a surgeon should be consulted, and they should be removed.

Occasionally the edges of the vulva are grown together at birth, thus completely occluding the opening. This condition is soon recognized and can be remedied by the physician. In other cases the closure is only partial and may not be discovered till marriage, when it is found that every attempt to accomplish the marital act is accompanied by intense pain. This can only be relieved by a surgical operation, and it should be attended to as soon as the condition is discovered.

Sometimes the orifice of the vagina is in a constant state of irritation, with a frequent desire to urinate, and severe pain and burning attending each passage of the urine. When such symptoms are present they indicate an irritation of the urethra or canal leading from the bladder, and an examination will often show one or more little groups or tumors at the mouth of this passage. These must be removed before any relief can be obtained.

INFLAMMATION OF THE VAGINA.

Inflammation of the Vagina may result from exposure to cold, injuries of any kind, the use of cold water and astringent injections to prevent conception, sexual excess, venereal poison, lack óf cleanliness and childbirth.

In such cases there is a severe itching of the vagina, accompanied by heat and burning, frequent desire to urinate, a smarting on passing the urine, and aching and dragging in the vagina, and around the anus (back passage), pain in lower part of abdomen and back, and a profuse yellowish discharge, with chaffing of the external parts, from the irritation of the poisonous discharges

Treatment.—The patient should remain in bed, and hot applications should be made to the vulva (privates) and lower part of the abdomen. The vagina should be cleansed by a full injection of hot water with a fountain syringe. If there is much pain an ounce of laudanum should be added to the injection. These injections should be used two or three times daily. When the acute symptoms have subsided, our H o m e Uterine Tablets should be used as directed till a cure is effected.

INFLAMMATION OF THE WOMB.

The womb, like other organs of the body, is liable to inflammation. It may affect the mucous membrane lining the womb, or it may involve all the structures of the womb, or may be confined to that part which extends into the vagina, called the neck of the womb.

From exposure to cold, direct injury (as a blow on the abdomen), or following miscarriage or childbirth, an acute inflammation may develop suddenly. In such cases there is intense pain in the region of the womb, which extends over the entire abdomen, burning heat in the vagina, and considerable general fever.

A chronic inflammation may remain after an acute attack, or may develop gradually as the result of some continued irritation, as excessive sexual indulgence, displacement of the womb, or laceration of the neck of the womb.

In these cases the patient complains of a dragging or bearing down sensation at the lower part of the abdomen, pain in the back and at the extreme end of the spine, and heaviness and dragging through the hips and thighs. There is also severe headache, especially on the top and back of the head; and as a rule there is considerable discharge from the vagina.

Treatment.—In acute inflammation of the womb the patient must remain quiet in bed, and hot applications must be made over the entire abdomen. Hot water douches given with a fountain syringe should be resorted to several times a day. To quiet the pain and relieve the fever our Neurodine Tablets should be given according to directions. When the acute symptoms subside the treatment for chronic inflammation may be necessary.

For chronic inflammation of the womb our Home Tonic Pills for Women should be used regularly for several months, or till all the symptoms above mentioned have disappeared. Warm water injections should be used to cleanse the vagina and one of our Home Uterine Tablets should be introduced, and repeated as directed on page 257. If this treatment is strictly followed, it will cure all cases that do not require surgical interference. Should it fail to cure, send for our "Question Blank for Women," and when we receive the answers to the questions, we will send a diagnosis of the case.

ULCERATION OF THE WOMB.

Ulceration of the Womb is a sequence of inflammation, and is often met with. The inflammation has extended to a breaking down of the tissues of the organ, and the formation of an ulcer, or sore. The symptoms are about the same as those of chronic inflammation, except that there is much more discharge from the vagina.

The home treatment is the same as that given for inflammation. When commenced as soon as the symptoms heretofore described are felt, the condition will be cured before it extends to ulceration. In long standing cases that do not yield to the treatment, some special course will be necessary.

LACERATION OF THE NECK OF THE WOMB.

The neck of the womb is often torn during childbirth, and thus keeps up a condition of chronic inflammation or ulceration. Sometimes the tare is very slight, but again it may be half an inch or even an inch in length. When this accident occurs it keeps up all the symptoms of chronic inflammation, in an aggravated form. The treatment above recommended for inflammation will relieve the symptoms, but will not cure them.

As many women have lacerated wombs without knowing it, they should be examined if the prescribed treatment does not effect a cure in a few months. An operation is the only thing that will insure a radical cure, and the sooner it is performed the better it will be for the patient.

DISPLACEMENTS OF THE WOMB.

The womb is liable to several forms of displacement, such as falling, tilting forward or backward, bending forward and backward on itself.

When these conditions are present the same general symptoms are felt as are present in other disorders of the womb. In addition, however, we often have a pressure on the bladder which causes a frequent desire to urinate, or a pressure on the rectum (back passage), which prevents natural actions of the bowels. In many cases the womb can be felt with the finger, within an inch or two from the orifice of the vagina. In many of these cases coitus is painful or even impossible, and conception cannot take place.

Chronic inflammation and enlargement of the womb are always present, and these conditions must be overcome by the treatment already recommended. Our H o m e Uterine Tablets act like a poultice in drawing the inflammation from the womb, and at the same time astringe the mucous surfaces, and contract the muscles of the vagina, thus forcing the womb up to its normal position. For this reason these tablets should be used for some time after all symptoms of inflammation have disappeared.

Some cases may require a mechanical support before a cure is effected, and this can only be applied by the experienced physician. No hard rubber or metal pessary should be used, and patients should avoid physicians who insist on such instruments being worn continuously.

LEUCORRHEA.

Leucorrhea, or Whites, is not a disease but a symptom of the several diseases of the vagina and womb, already described. It is a general term applied to any discharge from the vagina, and is often the first symptom that attracts attention. It is frequently so profuse as to be extremely annoying, and any woman suffering from it will hail with delight any remedy that will afford prompt relief from this unpleasant condition. Such a remedy is now within the reach of all. Our H o m e Uterine Tablets will arrest this discharge after the introduction of the first one, and will cure it entirely if used according to directions.

LACERATION OF THE PERINEUM.

The perineum is the space between the vagina and the rectum, and it supports the vagina, womb, bladder, and rectum, in their normal position. It is often torn through during childbirth. and if not properly attended to at the time it remains open, and thus removes the natural support from the organs named. As a result we have all the symptoms of inflammation and falling of the womb, and the woman soon becomes a confirmed invalid.

The only relief in such cases is to be had from an operation. When properly performed the parts are restored to their normal position, and all inflammation can then be readily overcome.

HYSTERIA.

Hysteria, or Hysterics. is a nervous condition to which women suffering from womb troubles are often liable. It is usually marked by extreme irritability of the nervous system, with mental depression. There is often a sensation of a lump in the throat, with muscular twitchings, which sometimes extend to extreme rigidity with partial loss of consciousness. At one moment the patient will laugh inordinately and will cry the next, without any apparent cause.

In all such cases the local conditions should be seen to, and the general system should be built up by the continued use of our H o m e Tonic Pills for Women.

ABSENCE OF CONJUGAL DESIRE.

It often happens that women who have suffered from diseases of the womb lose all desire for the conjugal act, and rarely have any enjoyment therefrom. When such a condition exists in those who have previously enjoyed such relations, it indicates some diseased condition of the generative organs, which can invariably be corrected. A physician should be consulted, and the patient should confide in him implicitly to insure a correction of the difficulty.

Some women have never enjoyed the marital act and are skeptical about their sisters doing so. In these cases there is usually some physical defect, either on her own part or on the part of the husband. It seldom happens that these conditions cannot be corrected, but a complete history of both husband and wife, as well as physical examinations are necessary to ascertain the cause or causes, and remedy the defect.

STERILITY, OR BARRENNESS.

All healthy women should be capable of bearing children, and yet thousands go through life longing for offspring who think themselves doomed to bar- renness.

There is always some recognizable cause for sterility in women, and it can almost invariably be corrected. Usually it can be traced to some disease or displacement of the womb, but in some cases the cause is a physiological one.

Consult an experienced physician and be guided by his advice, and a remedy for sterility can almost invariably be found.

TUMORS.

The womb and ovaries are frequently the seat of abnormal growths, or tumors. Those involving the womb are often attended by profuse flooding at every monthly period, and those of the ovaries us- ually attain a large size in a short time.

As soon as any indication of enlargement of the abdomen, or filling up of the vagina is manifest, a surgeon should be consulted, and the tumor should be removed at the earliest possible moment.

CANCER.

A Cancer is a malignant tumor, which is always certain to prove fatal in periods ranging from six months to two years, if not properly treated. It occurs most frequently in the breast and the womb. In the breast a hard lump forms, which gradually increases in size and soon causes a darting, shooting pain. A lump in the breast should always be regarded with suspicion, and as soon as it appears a surgeon should be consulted.

In the womb a cancer is attended with darting pains, frequent bleeding, and a very offensive discharge.

It is now generally conceded that cancer is at first a local disease, which becomes constitutional after the tumor has broken down so that the poison can be absorbed with the blood.

In genuine cancers, the treatment by plasters and caustics is never successful. The only rational and sure cure is an early removal of the diseased part, by a surgical operation. We have many cases where the patients are now enjoying perfect health fifteen and twenty years after the operation.

CHAPTER XIII.

The Eye and Its Disorders.

CARE OF THE EYES—DEFECTS OF VISION—THE USE
OF SPECTACLES—DISEASES OF THE LIDS—WEEP-
ING, OR WATERY, EYES—CROSS-EYE—CONJUNC-
TIVITIS—GRANULAR LIDS—ULCERATION OF THE
CORNEA—OPACITY OF THE CORNEA—IRITIS—
CATARACT—GLAUCOMA—AMAUROSIS.

The eye is one of the most important organs of
the body and through it, as the special organ of
sight we receive much of our knowledge of the
beauties of nature and the condition of things
around us.

It is withal the most perfect of optical instruments, but its functions are easily impaired or destroyed by any violation of natural laws.

It is seldom that people are born blind; but
blindness is invariably due to abuse of the eyes
by overwork and neglect, or improper treatment of
the several diseases and injuries of the eye.

Every one should know how to use the eyes
without abusing them, and should be able to deter-
mine for himself when there is need to use glasses;
and should also know enough of the nature of the

several diseases and deformities of the eye, to re-
alize the importance of consulting an oculist at the
earliest possible moment. Only a few brief suggestions on this important subject can be offered
in this manual, but it is to be hoped that these will
be heeded, and prove of value to many of our
readers.

THE CARE OF THE EYES.

The care of the eyes should begin with the new-
born babe. Carelessness in properly cleansing the
eyes immediately after birth often results in severe
inflammation which either destroys the sight in a
few days or weeks, or entails a life time of suffering
from weakness and defect of vision.

Reading on cars or in a dim light should be
avoided. The constant motion of the cars keeps
the book or paper jaring continuously, thus taxing
the eye to keep the proper focus, while the lack of
sufficient light causes the eyes to make extra efforts
to concentrate the vision.

The back or side should be toward the light
while reading or doing any close work. This lights
up the print or work, and does not allow too much
light to enter the eye, and thus contract the pupils.

Never rub the eyes when dust or cinders get
into them. Instead, close the eyes for a few moments, when the accumulated tears will wash the
foreign bodies toward the nose, when they can be
easily removed with a soft handkerchief or brush

pressed into the inner corner of the eye and carried toward the nose.

If hard substances, as pieces of steel, iron, or glass, are imbedded in the structures of the eye, motion should be prevented by means of a compress and bandage applied to the eye till a competent surgeon can be sent for.

When any caustic or burning substance, such as lime, cinders, acids, etc., gets into the eye, the lid should be held open and sweet olive oil or vaseline should be applied till an experienced surgeon can be consulted.

When the eye is injured in any way light should be excluded and motion prevented, by applying a loose bandage, till the surgeon arrives.

The eyes should never be used in reading or close work after a tired or strained feeling of the eyes is observed.

Whenever any defect of vision is recognized an oculist should be consulted with the view of having normal vision restored by properly adjusted spectacles.

DEFECTS OF VISION.

The several defects of vision are caused by changes in the shape of the eyeballs or the inability of the muscles to concentrate the eyes to a proper focus. These defects are known as myopia or near sight, hypermetropia or oversight, presbyopia or old sight, and astigmatism or irregular sight.

Myopia necessitates the bringing of all objects close to the eye to secure good vision. If this type cannot be seen till it is closer than eight inches to the eyes, the person must be near sighted. As soon as this condition is recognized in children, they should be examined, and have properly adjusted concave glasses to restore normal vision. This done and the eyes will increase in strength, and during early manhood the glasses may be entirely left aside.

Hypermetropia, or oversight, requires a constant straining effort to secure good vision, at normal distances; and this print must be carried farther than twelve inches from the eye to be seen distinctly. When used the eyes soon become tired and the vision blurred, and pain is felt in the balls of the eyes, and through the forehead. Convex glasses will entirely restore normal vision for both near and distant objects, and they should be worn as soon as any eye strain is felt.

Presbyopia, or old sight, always appears as age advances. It is manifested by a disposition to carry print farther from the eye than usual to secure good vision. When the sight begins to show a weakening in this way, convex glasses should be resorted to at once for reading or any close work. The longer the use of glasses is delayed, the weaker the eyes become, and thus much stronger glasses will be required to restore the vision.

Astigmatism, or irregular sight, is caused by irregularities in the shape of the globe of the eye, and thus an irregular image is formed in the eye, which causes a defect of vision. This condition may escape notice for a long time, and when recognized it is often found that the patient had never been able to see distinctly. It sometimes exists by itself, but is often present with near sight and oversight

These conditions require spectacles made specially for each case to restore normal vision.

THE USE OF SPECTACLES.

Many defects of vision exist from birth which require the use of spectacles. Others are caused by over taxation of the eye, by local injuries, and as the result of disease. Again normal vision begins to fail in most persons between the ages of thirty-five and fifty. Whatever may be the cause or the conditions present, all persons who find their vision defective should endeavor to correct the same by the proper use of glasses. Putting off the use of glasses as long as possible always does harm. They should be resorted to on the first indication of failing sight.

The following suggestions should be remembered by those whose sight is in any way defective.

First.—As soon as it is necessary to hold ordinary print further from the eyes than formerly an oculist should be consulted with the view of having glasses properly adjusted.

Second.—At first the glasses need only be used while reading or working by an artificial light.

Third.—If glasses magnify the letters when first worn they are two strong and should not be used.

Fourth.—Never buy cheap glasses, from pedlers or dry-goods stores, as they will do harm instead of good.

Fifth.—In old sight the glasses used for reading should never be used for distant vision.

Sixth.—A single eye-glass should never be used.

Seventh.—Spectacle frames should always be used instead of eye-glasses for any kind of continuous work requiring the constant use of the eyes.

DISEASES OF THE LIDS.

The eyelids are often the seat of disease and deformities which occasion great annoyance even when they do not injure the sight.

Small bunches or tumors sometimes form on the eyelids. They are caused by an obstruction of the minute ducts that open on the margin of the lids and supply a lubricant to the eyelashes. This causes the natural secretion to accumulate in the gland, thus forming the tumor.

Sometimes these little lumps will disappear by rubbing them with the finger several times a day; but if they do not, the sack containing the accumu-

lation should be removed by making an opening
on the inside of the lid.

Small pustules, or boils, often form on the margin of the lid, and are popularly known as "stys."
They commence as a small inflamed spot and gradually pus or matter is formed. When they occur
they should be opened with a new needle that has
been previously washed in boiling water, and then
the matter can be gently pressed out. In ordinary
cases no further treatment is necessary; but when
one sty follows another in rapid succession, our
H o m e Sarsaparilla Pills should be used to purify
the blood.

When the eyelashes are bent in so as to press
against the ball of the eye, or when there is a
double row of lashes, the eye is kept in a constant
state of inflammation.

Pulling out the inverted lashes by the roots with
a pair of pliers will give temporary relief, but a
specialist should be consulted for a complete cure.

Sometimes the lid is turned outward so that its
inner surface is exposed to view, and again the lid
is turned in so that the lashes and skin rest against
the ball of the eye. In both these conditions an
oculist should be consulted at once, as the eye will
become permanently injured if the deformity is not
corrected.

Drooping of the eyelid is a condition of paralysis
of the upper lid which makes it impossible to raise
the lid by voluntary effort. This can be relieved

by a simple operation, which should be performed as soon as possible, in order to preserve the sight.

WEEPING, OR WATERY, EYES.

This is a condition where there is an obstruction in the canal that carries the tears from the eye to the cavity of the nose. This causes the tears to accumulate in the inner corner of the eye till they flow over the margin of the lower lid and down the cheeks. Sometimes an abscess will form between the angle of the eye and the nose. If neglected this condition soon weakens the eye and dims the vision.

A simple operation is necessary to relieve the obstruction, but to insure the success of the operations probes must be inserted daily for some time, to dilate the canal and prevent it from closing again.

CROSS-EYE.

By Cross-eye is meant a turning in or out of one or both eyes in such a manner as to prevent the use of both eyes in looking at an object. It is usually acquired during infancy by placing the child so that it can only see with one eye; but is frequently caused by the nervous irritation which accompanies teething, whooping cough, measles, scarlet fever, and convulsions.

To correct this deformity a simple operation is required, and it should be performed as soon as possible after the condition is noticed. If delayed the vision of one or both eyes is liable to be impaired.

CONJUNCTIVITIS.

Conjunctivitis is an inflammation of a thin membrane that covers the ball of the eye and lines the eye lids. It is commonly called an inflamed eye.

It may result from cold, slight injury, the presence in the eye of foreign bodies, and the contact of poisonous matter.

The eye becomes red and swollen, the flow of tears is increased, and it becomes intolerant of light.

Treatment.—If there is any foreign body in the eye it should be removed at once, and the eye should be bathed in water as hot as can be borne. Then one of our H o m e Eye Tablets should be dissolved in an eye-bath full of tepid water, and the eye should be thoroughly bathed with this three or four times a day. This treatment will also radically cure all cases of chronically inflamed eyes, where no granulation of the lids is present.

GRANULATED LIDS.

Granulated lids is a condition of chronic inflammation of the conjunctivita. The lids are very much thickened and their under surfaces are covered by minute little elevations, called granulations, which become hard and cause an irritation of the front part of the ball of the eye, which is called the cornea. If this condition is neglected it soon causes a loss of sight.

In these and all long-standing inflammations of the eyes, the patient should place himself under the personal care of an experienced surgeon.

ULCERATION OF THE CORNEA.

The cornea is the clear, transparent front part of the eye, through which the light passes to the interior of the eye.

It is sometimes the seat of inflammation which may extend to ulceration. This is an eating into the tissues of the cornea, and if neglected it may penetrate the cornea, and thus destroy the sight.

All these cases require the constant care of the surgeon, and home treatment should not be attempted.

OPACITY OF THE CORNEA.

This is a condition resulting from inflammation and ulceration of the cornea. It begins by a hazy film forming over the outer surface of the cornea, which dims the vision. This gradually increases till a thick white film covers the entire front of the eye, and totally destroys the sight. It is sometimes spoken of as "external cataract," and it is even confounded with cataract.

The majority of cases of opacity of the cornea can be cured if properly treated; but the treatment must be under the immediate supervision of a surgeon.

IRITIS.

The iris is the dark circular membrane that surrounds the pupil.

It is liable to inflammation which is called Iritis. When it occurs there is considerable pain in the eye, and the pupil becomes irregular in shape, and after a time it may be entirely obliterated, thus destroying the sight. This disease should be treated by an experienced surgeon, and even when sight is lost, it can be restored by an operation.

CATARACT.

By Cataract is meant an opacity of a small body in the interior of the eye, called the crystalline lens, or of a thin membrane which covers it. This lens plays an important part in the production of vision, as it brings the rays of light to a focus on the retina, to produce the image of the object looked at in the eye.

This lens is transparent, like glass, but in this disease it becomes clouded and finally perfectly white or yellowish, so as to exclude light entirely.

An operation is the only means of restoring sight in cases of cataract. This consists in removing the opaque lens from the eye, and after the eye has entirely healed, the defect is supplied by powerful convex glasses. The operation should be performed as soon as vision is destroyed, and none but an experienced surgeon should undertake it.

GLAUCOMA.

This is an inflammatory condition that involves all the tissues and contents of the eyeball. It progresses rapidly, and soon completely destroys the sight. It is recognized by a sense of fullness and pressure of the eye, which feels as if the ball would burst. An operation, if performed in time, will sometimes save the sight.

AMAUROSIS.

This term indicates a gradual loss of sight, and usually comes on after diseases of the brain or nervous prostration. It is due to some impairment of the functions of the optic nerve, and as a rule it is not amenable to treatment.

CHAPTER XIV.

The Ear and Its Disorders.

CARE OF THE EARS—MALFORMATIONS AND INJURIES OF THE EARS—ACCUMULATION OF WAX—ABSCESS—POLYPUS—DEAFNESS.

The ear is the organ of the special sense of hearing, and is described by anatomists as being divided into the external, middle, and internal ear. The broad expansion on the side of the head, which is commonly called the ear, serves to collect the vibrations of the atmosphere and convey them to the opening of the canal that leads to the " drum of the ear." This canal is called the external auditory canal, and that with the broad expansion constitutes the *external ear.*

The inner terminus of this canal is closed by a thin movable membrane called the " drum of the ear," the movements of which play an important part in the production of sound.

The middle ear is a small chamber situated in the temporal bone, which contains a little chain of three small bones which move upon each other when pressed on by the " drum of the ear," and thus convey a vibration to the internal ear. The middle ear in health contains air, which enters it through a canal leading from the throat, called the eustachian tube.

The internal ear is composed of a number of canals and shell-like cavities, on the inner surfaces of which are distributed the minute filaments of the auditory nerve—the special nerve of hearing.

When sound is produced, the waves of air strike the "drum of the ear" and press it inward so as to move the chain of bones in the middle ear. The third bone moves upon the opening of the internal ear, and causes a motion of the liquid it contains. This motion is received by the filaments of the auditory nerve and is then conveyed to the brain, where it produces a sensation called sound.

It is necessary that the eustachian tube should be free to admit air to the middle ear, for otherwise the "drum" would not move, and no sound could be produced.

Any disturbance of the normal condition of these parts causes an impairment or entire loss of hearing. It is therefore important that every person should know how to care for the ear so as to prevent deafness.

CARE OF THE EARS.

A perfectly healthy ear requires no special care. The wax dries up in thin scales and comes away gradually and imperceptibly, while all attempts to keep the ear clean with brushes, **ear** sponges, etc., will certainly do harm.

It will be well to observe the following simple rules, in order to keep the ears in a healthy state.

First.—Avoid washing the ears with soap and water, or using brushes, sponges, or a screwed-up corner of a towel; but cleans it while washing, only as far as can be reached with the finger.

Second.—Never use earpicks or pins, as they always cause irritation.

Third.—Do not, as a rule, cover the ears in cold weather, except when exposed to a severe storm.

Fourth.—When slight deafness accompanies a severe cold, it indicates a closure of the eustachian tube at its orifice in the throat, and efforts should be made at once to reduce the inflammation and soreness of the throat.

Fifth.—The constant dropping into the **ear** of strong medicines, oils, or glycerine, should be avoided unless recommended by a competent surgeon.

Sixth.—Parents should never strike a child on the ear or head, as such violence may rupture the " drum of the ear " and cause deafness.

Seventh.—When a child complains of pain in the ears it should be seen to at once; and, in the absence of advice from a physician, hot applications to the external ear should be used till the doctor comes.

Eighth.—Discharges from the **ear** after scarlet

fever, measles, etc., should be attended to at once, as permanent deafness may result from neglect.

Ninth.—When insects or any foreign bodies get into the ear, they can be removed by injecting warm water, with a common ear syringe; but ear-picks and forcepts should never be used.

Tenth.—Cold water should never be introduced into the ear. While bathing the ear should be protected by filling the external opening with cotton before going into the water.

MALFORMATION AND INJURIES.

Malformations of the external ear are often present at birth, and the ear may be wounded by blows, and torn by wearing heavy ear-rings. These conditions require the attention of a surgeon, and simple operations can be performed to entirely correct these conditions.

ACCUMULATION OF WAX.

Sometimes there is an excessive secretion of wax in the ear, which accumulates in a hard lump and finally fills the entire external auditory canal.

This gives rise to noises in the head, dizziness, deafness, and inflammation of the canal.

A surgeon should be consulted for the removal of this wax and the treatment of the inflamed canal, and above all the use of pins and earpricks must be avoided, or injury of the ear may be caused.

ABSCESS OF THE EAR.

Abscesses often form in the ears, as a result of inflammation caused by taking cold or injury to the ear. They are very painful while the condition lasts, but are not dangerous. The pain is of a deep-seated beating, throbbing character, and it may extend to the entire side of the face. It subsides, however, as soon as pus (matter) forms, and stops entirely when the abscess breaks. While it lasts the hearing is impaired.

Hot fomentations of hops or hot poultices should be applied to the ear till a physician can be sent for. It is always best that the doctor should open the abscess as soon as the throbbing pain is felt, as a free incision relieves the congested part and cuts short the suffering.

POLYPUS.

A Polypus is a small tumor that develops in the external canal, and so fills it up that deafness is produced.

When a polypus is present there is an offensive discharge from the ear, noises in the head, and sometimes severe pain. If the ear is examined, in a good light, the polypus can be seen like a small fleshy body filling up the canal.

In all such cases a surgeon should be consulted, and the polypus should be removed at once, as it is liable to destroy the " drum of the ear," and thus cause permanent deafness.

DEAFNESS.

Deafness may result from a great variety of causes, and a careful examination by an experienced surgeon is necessary for a correct diagnoses. In all cases, except those where the optic nerve is paralyzed or the " drum " is destroyed, the hearing can be improved or entirely restored, and even these cases can be benefitted.

No case of deafness should be long neglected, but a surgeon should be consulted, and the cause removed at the earliest possible moment.

CHAPTER XV.

Surgical Diseases and Accidents.

PILES — FISTULA OF THE ANUS — FISSURE OF THE ANUS—HERNIA, OR RUPTURE—VARICOSE VEINS — INGROWN TOE NAILS — DISEASES OF THE BONES— FRACTURES— SPRAINS— DISLOCATIONS —DISEASES OF THE JOINTS—SPINAL DEFORMITIES — KNOCK KNEE — BOWED LEGS — CLUB FOOT—ULCERS—TUMORS--CANCERS.

A description of the several surgical diseases and accidents would fill many large volumes; and brief references to a few of them are given here only with the hope that sufferers may recognize the conditions early, and thus be ennabled to obtain relief before the more serious complications are developed.

PILES.

Hemorrhoids, or piles, is an enlarged condition of the veins of the rectum, caused by constipation, torpid liver, exposure to cold, the pressure of a displaced womb, rectal tumors, continued diarrhea, and the action of powerful purgative medicines.

This condition rarely develops before the age of

puberty, but is very common among adults of both sexes. It is estimated that one person in ten suffers from some form of piles.

There are two varieties of the disease, viz., external and internal piles.

The external pile begins as a lump at the verge of the anus, which rapidly fills with blood, and becomes hard and painful. It can be felt with the finger, and presents a bluish appearance.

The internal pile is situated inside of the bowel, and begins with an itching burning sensation, and a feeling of fullness and weight in the rectum. Pain is felt with every action of the bowels, and sometimes the passage is seriously obstructed. Bleeding will often occur with each movement of the bowels, and then the condition is spoken of as bleeding piles.

When the enlargement attains a considerable size, the pile is forced through the constricting muscles, and protrudes beyond the anus, and is then called protruding piles. When this condition occurs, the muscles often contract so as to constrict the protruding mass, thus occasioning marked swelling and intense pain.

Only one tumor appears in some cases, while in others there may be a cluster of three or four.

Treatment.—The external pile is the most speedily relieved by having a surgeon open the vein and squeeze out the clotted blood. This gives immediate relief, while the application of our H o m e Pile

Ointment will rapidly heal the part and contract the vein, so as to prevent a recurrence of the trouble.

Internal piles may be paliated or relieved by bathing the parts in hot water, and applying our Home Pile Ointment, well up the rectum with the finger, two or three times a day. The bowels must be kept regular by the use of our Home Liver Pills, and the patient should keep off his feet for a few days as much as possible. When a person has once had an attack of piles he is almost certain to have a recurrence at some time, and each attack is likely to be more severe than the preceeding ones. When they once begin to protrude they are certain to occasion great annoyance, and the only sure relief is an operation for a radical cure.

There are several methods of operating on piles, but none but an experienced surgeon should be trusted to operate. We have operated on thousands of cases during the past thirty years without a single failure. To those desiring information regarding our method of treatment, we will send full particulars on receipt of a full description of their cases.

FISTULA OF THE ANUS

A fistula of the anus is an unnatural canal that extends up some distance by the side of the rectum, and almost constantly discharges matter. It may open through the skin and into the bowel, when it is called a complete fistula; it may open through the skin only, when it is called an external blind fistula;

or it may open into the bowel alone, when it is called an internal blind fistula.

It may be caused by an abscess near the anus, or by an ulceration of the rectum eating through the coats of the bowels into the surrounding tissue.

There is always a discharge of matter either from the bowel or the external opening, but at times it may be very slight, and then again very profuse. There is a feeling of tenderness and soreness about the part, and sometimes sharp pains.

An operation is the only means by which a cure can be effected, and the sooner this is performed the better for the patient. A radical cure can always be guaranteed when a proper operation is performed.

FISSURE OF THE ANUS.

A fissure of the anus is a crack or split in the mucous surface, extending from inside the bowel downward beyond the verge of the anus. It soon assumes the appearance of an ulcer, from which an acrid discharge is thrown off, which irritates and chafes the surrounding parts. Each passage from the bowels causes a stretching and scratching sensation, which will soon arrest the normal action, and cause constipation.

This is another condition that requires the attention of a surgeon, as an operation is the only thing that will insure a radical cure.

HERNIA, OR RUPTURE.

Hernia, or Rupture, as generally used, means a protrusion of a fold of the bowel through a weak point in the walls of the abdomen. It occurs in both sexes, and it is claimed that one person in seven is affected by it.

If left protruding it is liable, at any time, to become inflamed and cause death. It is, therefore, necessary to force the protruding bowel back to its place, and prevent it from coming out again. The usual means of accomplishing this is by wearing a truss, which is so constructed as to keep up sufficient pressure at the weak point, to prevent the bowel from protruding.

Many persons, however, find it difficult to get a truss that will hold up the rupture, while most people find the truss very uncomfortable.

Modern surgery has come to the aid of such sufferers, and now an operation can be performed that will insure a radical cure in two or three weeks. Full particulars of the operation will be sent on application.

VARICOSE VEINS.

By Varicose Veins is meant an enlarged and twisted condition of the veins of the extremities. Such conditions are accompanied by a feeling of weight of the extremities, with more or less pain, after any exertion.

The use of elastic stockings will give support to

the part and afford considerable comfort, but an operation is necessary for a cure.

INGROWN TOE NAILS.

This is a condition where the side of the toe nail grows down into the flesh, thus causing an irritation, which often extends to inflammation and ulceration. It seldom involves any but the great toes, and usually occasions much suffering.

If the ingrowing side of the nail is carefully raised up and cut off with a sharp pair of scissors or knife, and then a piece of cotton saturated with a solution of persulphate of iron crowded under the edge, great relief is obtained at once. The application of the iron on the cotton can be repeated every two or three days, till the edge of the nail seems dry and shrivelled. The growth of the nail will be arrested in this way and a cure is effected.

If this cannot be done, a simple operation can be performed which will permanently relieve the trouble.

DISEASES OF THE BONES.

The bones are liable to inflammation, ulceration, and death, as a result of injuries and constitutional defects. The parts affected become hot, swollen, and painful, and the use of the extremity involved is seriously impaired. After a time, matter forms and openings along the bone are produced for its escape. If this does not occur blood-poisoning may

result. If neglected these openings will continue
to discharge unhealthy matter, mixed with small
pieces of bone, and will permanently destroy the
usefulness of the limb.

Such cases should never be neglected but should
be placed under the care of an experienced surgeon.
The proper operation will arrest the further destruction of the bone, and favor the production of new
bone.

FRACTURES.

Fractures, or broken bones, are so easily recognized as the result of injuries, that no description
of them is necessary. It is always important that
the existence of a fracture should be recognized as
soon as it occurs, and that the bones should be
properly adjusted and held in position till a union
has taken place. With this end in view a surgeon
should be sent for at once, and when the dressings
are once applied, neither the patient nor his friends
should interfere with them.

SPRAINS.

A sprain is a wrench or twist of a joint by which
the ligaments are stretched or torn, without a fracture or dislocation.

A severe sprain is often more annoying than a
fracture, and the person suffering from one should
at once desist from using the injured joint.

If it can be attended to before inflammation sets

in, cold applications will be found very serviceable. If, however, some hours have elapsed before anything is done, hot applications, as hot fomentations of hops will serve the best purpose. Absolute rest of the injured joint is imperative, and when an attempt is made to use it, after all inflammation and swelling have subsided, a tight bandage should be applied to give the support,

DISLOCATIONS.

By dislocation is meant a forcible separation of the bones that form a joint. It is always produced by violence of some kind; and whenever a joint is injured a competent surgeon should be sent for, so that the displacement can be recognized and overcome before inflammation and swelling set in.

DISEASES OF THE JOINTS.

The several joints of the body are liable to be affected by inflammation, which may be confined to a particular part or may involve all the structures of the joint.

The inflammation may come on suddenly, when it is attended by pain, heat, redness, and swelling of the joints; or it may develop gradually and even escape notice for a considerable time after the disease has set in. It may result from a direct local injury, from exposure to cold or damp, and from blood poisoning.

As soon as a joint becomes painful and begins

to swell it should be kept entirely quiet, and a surgeon should be sent for.

When the inflammation assumes a chronic form,
the tissues of the joint may be entirely destroyed,
and deformity and permanent stiffness may result.
For this reason proper treatment must be had as
soon as possible, so as to insure the extension and
fixation of the joint, which will alone insure a radical cure.

In many cases of hip-joint disease, the first
symptoms are a slight stiffness of the joint, a disposition to stand on one foot, a limping gait, pain
on the inner side of the knee, and tenderness on
pressure over the joint. When these symptoms
are noticed, especially in a child, the patient
should be placed on his back with the legs extended. Then a quick blow is made on the sole of the
foot, with sufficient force to move the entire leg.
If sharp pain is felt in the hip joint, it will be a
sure indication that the joint is affected, and it
should be attended to without delay.

When a severe inflammation sets in from the
start in this joint, it is liable to run its course rapidly, and result in the formation of matter and the
destruction of the head of the bone in a very short
time.

In all such cases a surgeon should be consulted
without delay.

Anchylosis, or stiffness of a joint, is liable to result from any inflammatory condition, and if the

joint is not properly moved in time, the stiffness may become permanent and thus destroy the use-'fulness of the limb.

'When such stiffness exists, the proper treatment will restore the motion in the majority of cases; but only a skillful surgeon should be intrusted with the case.

SPINAL DEFORMITIES.

As a result of injury, constitutional weakness, and unnatural positions in sitting, children frequently develop deformities of the spinal column, or back bone.

When the bodies of the bones of the spine are diseased and the weight of the upper part of the body causes a backward curving of the spine, it is called Pott's disease, or backward curvature, and when the spine is twisted sideways it is called lateral curvature.

Whichever condition develops, a pronounced deformity is soon produced, which keeps increasing, so as to prevent the child from growing tall, and often results in death.

When the proper treatment is neglected protruding shoulders and back are the result, and the patient goes through life crippled and deformed.

These cases were formerly treated by steel braces, with thumb screws and springs to press upon the protruding parts. Such appliances do more harm than good, and should never be worn.

The proper treatment consists of extending the spine, so as to lift the weight of the body off the deformed spine, and then applying something to support this weight off the diseased bones. This is best done by the application of the plaster of Paris jacket. When properly applied it gives immediate relief, can be worn with comfort, and is certain to result in a radical cure in the hands of an experienced surgeon.

We have treated hundreds of cases, of all varieties, of spinal troubles by this method and have never failed of a cure when the patients have followed directions. The treatment requires great patience and care on the part of the surgeon, and persistence on the part of the patient.

KNOCK KNEE.

By Knock Knee is meant a spreading apart of the legs below the knee, and a knocking of the knees against each other while walking. It is a deformity of early childhood, which becomes a serious deformity if neglected.

As soon as the condition is noticed a surgeon should be consulted and a proper instrument should be applied to overcome the deformity before the bones become hardened. .

BOWED LEGS.

Bowed Legs result from a bending outwards of the legs so that the knees are far apart, and the legs are arched like a bow. The condition is generally caused by allowing children to stand before the bones of the legs have become sufficiently hardened to support the weight of the body.

This deformity should be corrected in childhood, and can be readily done by the application of the proper apparatus.

CLUB FOOT.

Club Foot is a deformity in which the foot is drawn from its natural position by muscular contraction. It is usually present at birth though it may sometimes be produced, during childhood, by injury to some of the muscles of the foot. There are several varieties of club foot and, if not corrected before the child begins to walk, a permanent deformity is sure to result The necessary operation is certain to overcome the difficulty, if properly performed and followed by the use of proper appliances to keep the foot in its normal position.

ULCERS.

An ulcer is an open sore where the skin and underlaying tissues have been destroyed as a result of severe inflammation. When it first develops and pain, heat and redness, are present, it is called an acute ulcer; but when it is of long standing, and the skin surrounding it assumes a dark purple color, and resists the usual efforts to heal, it is called a chronic ulcer.

Old ulcers are more frequently met with on the legs, below the knees, than anywhere else, but they may occur on any part of the body. They usually discharge an unhealthy pus, and cause the patient much annoyance.

Many people have an idea that an old ulcer should not be healed, as they think it is intended to remove impurities from the body, which would be deposited elsewhere if the ulcer is healed. It is needless to say that this is an old fogy idea which has no foundation in fact. Any person suffering from an old ulcer should consult a surgeon at once, and when the proper treatment is employed, even the worst cases can be cured in a short time. The part must first be stimulated by hot poultices for two or three days, and then antiseptic dressings should be employed, and the patient must keep entirely quiet, as motion always retards the healing process.

TUMORS.

Tumors are abnormal growths, and may be entirely new formations or excessive development of the structures of any part or organ of the body. They vary in size and shape according to their character and location. Some are not larger than a grain of wheat, while others attain enormous proportions.

Surgical writers divide tumors into two general classes, viz., benign and malignant. A benign tumor is one that does not disturb the general health or endanger life, except when it attains a size that will cause pressure on some important vessel or organ, while a malignant tumor is one that will of itself cause death in a short time. The latter form of tumors are popularly called cancers, and will be described below.

There are a number of varieties of benign tumors, the more common being, fatty, encysted, fibrous, and bony. When they occur they are usually situated where they produce deformity or cause inconvenience; and as soon as recognized, a surgeon should be consulted with the view of removal, especially if they show a tendency to grow rapidly.

CANCERS.

Cancers are more properly called malignant tumors. They may occur in any portion of the body, but are more frequently met with in the female breast and womb. See page 176.

There are several varieties of cancer, the more common being scirrhus or hard cancer; encepheloid or soft cancer, and epithelial cancer.

The hard cancer begins as a hard lump, which soon develops darting, shooting pains. They are movable at first but gradually become adherent to the surrounding tissues. The glands next become involved and the blood becomes poisoned, and death ensues in from eighteen months to two years.

Soft cancer develops more rapidly, has less pain,

and often bleeds freely after it breaks down. It may terminate in from six to eighteen months.

Epithelial cancer develops on the lips and at other outlets of the body where the skin and mucous surfaces join. This form is less fatal than the other varieties, and runs a much longer course.

It is now generally acknowledged that cancers begin as the result of local injuries, when the system is not in condition to supply healthy material to repair the injuries, and that a degeneration of tissue takes place, which in time is absorbed into the blood, and produces constitutional poisoning.

Whenever a hard lump is found accompanied by pain, or where there is a crack or ulcer on the lip, or other part of the body, that refuses to heal, an experienced surgeon should be consulted at once, and if a cancer is suspected no time should be lost in having it removed.

When removed before it breaks down and becomes an open sore, a cure can be safely assured, and at this stage the knife is the only safe and radical method of treatment. Plasters and caustics often remove non-malignant tumors, which are ignorantly called cancers, but in a genuine cancer they invariably do harm. The reason that cancers recur so often after the use of the knife is that the operation is usually delayed till the poison enters the system, when it is too late for any treatment to be of any avail.

On the other hand when plasters are used in the

early stages of cancer, they hasten the breaking down of the growth, and the poisoning of the system.

An early and thorough extirpation of the entire diseased part is the only safe course to adopt in a l cases of cancer.

CHAPTER XVI.

Food in Health and Disease.

INFANT FEEDING—FOOD FOR ADULT LIFE—FOOD IN
OLD AGE—FALLACIES REGARDING EATING—
DIET IN DYSPEPSIA—FOOD IN BILIOUSNESS—
FOOD IN NERVOUS ᐧ PROSTRATION — FOOD IN
RHEUMATISM—FOOD IN DIABETES—FOOD IN
CONSUMPTION — DIET IN ACUTE DISEASES —
FOOD IN CONVALESCENCE.

The human body is made up of a number of
elementary substances which exist in the form of
compounds within the body. These compounds
are called proximate principles by physiologists,
and this term is meant to designate the form in
which the elements exist in the body. These elements are constantly being used up and thrown off
by the vital processes as effete material, and in order to keep up the vital action their places must be
supplied by new material from without. The
source of supply is obtained from the food, which
undergoes proper digestion, and is then distributed
to the various parts of the body to nourish the tissues and supply the place of the waste material

that has been thrown off, and also to sustain animal life. It will therefore be seen that food should contain all the substances of which the body is composed.

The study of the anatomy of the organs of digestion demonstrates the fact that the human digestive apparatus is designed for the digestion of both animal and vegetable foods, and all attempts to make it appear that man should live on an exclusively vegetable diet have proved fallacies, and are contrary to the laws of nature.

Foods are divided into two classes: *First*—The hydro-carbons, or those that contain the elements of carbon, oxygen, and hydrogen. These serve to keep up animal heat, and embrace all starches, sugars and fats. *Second*—Albumenoids, or those that contain nitrogen in addition to the carbon, oxygen, and hydrogen, and which constitute the substances that go to build up tissue. In addition to these water makes up a large portion of the human body, and consequently a large quantity of this fluid must be taken into the system as part of the diet. Again there are a number of salts or earthy materials, such as common salt and the different forms of lime, that are essential to make up the different tissues and fluids of the body. When these are not found in combination with the articles of food, it is necessary that they should be supplied as such, either with the food or as medicine. The hydro-carbons, or heat producing foods, include all the cereals used

as the food of man, such as wheat, oats, barley, corn
and rye, and such vegetables as potatoes, peas,
beans, lentils, rice, tapioca, arrowroot, beets, carrots, parsnips, turnips, etc., and sugars of all kinds.
In addition to these all fats and oils properly belong
to this class, though they differ from the others in
containing more carbon and less oxygen.

The albumenoids include milk, cheese, eggs,
meats of all kinds, and the gluten of the cereals.

A healthy person in the prime of life will, as a
rule, enjoy the best health when due attention is
paid to a proper admixture of these foods, as the
starches and sugars are essential to supply the heat
necessary to keep up animal life, while the meats,
etc., give the strength and vitality that comes of
building up the tissues.

For the sake of convenience, however, life might
properly be divided into three periods: *First*—The
period of development or growth; *Second*—Adult
life; *Third*—Old age, or decay.

From the birth of the child until its eighteenth
or twenty-first year, the organs of the body are constantly developing. In fact growth begins at the
very birth of the child, and at that time when
there is little motion or muscular effort required,
the food should be composed largely of the
elements requisite for building up tissue. Hence
the first food for an infant as supplied by nature is
mother's milk, which is composed of water, albumenoid substances, and some fat and sugar. The

tissue building greatly exceeds the heat-producing ingredients in milk, and thus the child grows rapidly as long as the milk is continued. Following out this provision of nature, when the child begins to take other food than the mother's milk the tissue-building foods should be greatly in excess of the heat-producing, hence the necessity of withholding from the child bread, potatoes, sugar, and vegetables in general. Its first food after the mother's milk should be animal broths and the juice of rare beef and mutton. These foods, with milk, should constitute the diet. When starchy foods and sugars are freely given they cannot be digested, and they simply remain in the stomach or intestines, causing fermentation and the consequent formation of gases, which irritates the stomach and bowels. In this way many children are affected with serious derangements of digestion, the most common of which is cholera morbus, or summer complaint, which in the majority of cases proves fatal. This condition could be entirely averted if proper attention was paid to the feeding of children after weaning.

An infant should be fed every two hours for the first six or eight months of its life, and after that about once in every three hours till it is two years old. From the second to the fourteenth year of age the diet of childhood demands close attention. Coffee, tea, wine, beer, and all exciting drinks, should be avoided, and the food should consist of succulent meats without condiments, eggs, oatmeal, bread, and potatoes, in moderation; baked apples, butter, farinaceous puddings, and milk. Young children should have at least four meals a day, and they should be carefully watched that they do not overload their stomach. During this time children are usually very active, and require the starchy and sugary food to produce animal heat, which is not so essential before the age of two years. After fourteen years of age a generous mixed diet should be supplied to children, as the more permanent and rapid growth takes place between that time and twenty-one years of age. Meats, beans, peas, lentils, gluten bread, etc., should constitute the larger portion of the diet, as the tissues are formed rapidly during that time.

INFANT FEEDING.

A newly born babe should not be fed before it is applied to the breast, a teaspoonful of water being all that should be given. It is a mistaken idea to think that a babe will starve before the mother's breast will secrete the milk. At the first application of the child to the breast it draws out a watery substance which seems to be necessary to give the proper stimulus to the stomach and bowels to cause the latter to move. Even if the milk should not come for two or three days, it is best to allow the child to wait until it is secreted, but the child should be put regularly to the breast, even though no milk is present. Mothers should not resort to the use of ale and beer to increase the flow of milk, for, instead of having the effect desired, it simply increases the watery portions of the milk, thus reducing its nutritive properties.

When a mother is healthy and has a goodly secretion of milk, no child should be weaned until it is at least a year old; but after its sixth month, broths and soups, without vegetables, or a piece of beef or mutton to suck may be given without doing harm. Good cow's milk may also be given after the sixth month if it seems that the child is not sufficiently nourished from the mother's milk.

In cases where a mother cannot nurse her child a good substitute for human milk is good cow's milk prepared as follows: The milk should be allowed to stand for an hour, after which the cream should be skimmed from the top. During the first month, four parts of this skimmed milk should be added to one part of water, and this sweetened by a few grains of sugar of milk. After the first month the same proportion of water should be added, but it is best to leave the cream with the milk; and after the second month ordinary cow's milk may be given pure.

A perfect food for infants and children must contain practically the same proportion of constituents and be as easily digested as a good quality of human milk, and when it is found impossible to use the breast milk, my personal experience shows that Carnrick's Soluble Food is the best in the market. It is also of great value as an Invalid Food, where other nutrients cannot be tolerated.

It is always best when a child is fed artificially that the milk should not be heated as is usually the case. It should stand for an hour in the living room of the child before using it. By adopting this course there is no possibility of having the milk too hot at one time and too cold at another, which varying conditions of temperature always have a bad effect upon the stomach of the child. After the sixth month animal broths and beef juice may be added to the diet, the same as previously recommended. As infants and young children will eat as long as they have anything before them, care should be taken to avoid this tendency to overloading the stomach, and should milk come up from the stomach as soon as swallowed it is an indication that the stomach is full and the child should at once be taken from the breast or the bottle. It is never a good plan to offer children food when they are restless or crying, unless two hours have elapsed since the previous feeding.

These precautions will save the child from having derangement of the stomach or bowels, and in all cases where they are observed there is much less liability of the children suffering from summer complaint.

FOOD FOR ADUDT LIFE.

After twenty-one years of age, as a rule, all the organs and tissues of the body are fully developed, and if healthy their functions are perfect. At this time the office of food is to keep up animal heat and to supply the waste of tissue. A generous mixed diet of both animal and vegetable food is essential to this period of maturity. The activity dependent upon the various pursuits of life not only demands a considerable supply of fuel to keep the machinery in motion, but also requires sufficient material to repair the waste that is constantly going on in the brain, muscles, nerves, and other tissues of the body. Here the quantity of the heat-producing and tissue-building foods are more evenly balanced, and it is important to know the relative values of the several foods for the respective purposes. Of the vegetables, those that contain the most starch, or the best heat-producing foods, contain the least amount of material necessary for tissue-building, as may be seen by the following examples: two pounds of wheat flour contain about one ounce of tissue-forming material; two pounds of turnips contain about one and one-half ounces; two pounds of potatoes contain about one ounce; and four pounds of carrots about one ounce; while one pound of oatmeal contains thirteen ounces. Cocoa nibs, dried beans, and peas, stand next to the oatmeal in the value of these substances. It will thus be seen that if a person abstains from eating meat, lentils, beans and peas, cocoa nibs and gluten bread supply the greatest amount of material for building-tissue, while they also contain a sufficient amount of starch to keep up the animal heat. But as considerable quantities of these things are necessary to take the place of a small quantity of roast beef or mutton, the animal foods are preferable as diet.

It is claimed by many that brain-workers require to eat large quantities of food containing phosphates, on the supposition that an extra amount of phosphates taken into the system are needed to supply the waste of brain-tissue. As science has proved, however, that phosphates exist in larger proportions in the muscles than in the brain, it does not follow that any special phosphatic food is necessary for brain-workers. It may be laid down as a rule that the brain-worker who eats a proper proportion of beef and mutton, with an admixture of ordinary vegetables, providing he rests long enough after eating to favor proper digestion, will find his brain in better working condition than the man who depends upon fish, oysters, and other so called phosphatic foods. In fact there is no fish except salmon that contains as much phosphatic material as beef or mutton, and the old notion that raw oysters are composed largely of phosphates has been shown to be a fallacy. It must be admitted, however, that very often a light meal of raw oysters is better for a brain-worker than roast beef and vegetables. This is due to the fact, however, that as raw oysters contain a large amount of pepsin they are very easily digested, and where a person is applying the mind very closely he is apt to begin his work so soon after eating that the blood is at once brought to the brain from the stomach, and thus digestion is impossible. This results in a short time in a chronic state of indigestion which of necessity prevents a proper nutrition of the body.

FOOD IN OLD AGE.

After fifty or fifty-five years of age, the nutritive process becomes less active. Even though there may be considerable activity of the mind and body, the amount of food consumed is usually much less than during the prime of life. The heat-producing foods should now be supplied in such forms as to render them most easy of digestion. Care should be given to the proper cooking of food, and mastication is likely to be imperfect. Meats should be chopped fine before broiling, that they may be more easily digested after swallowing. Milk at this period often constitutes an important article of diet, even though it may not have been much used during the prime of life.

The question of stimulants now comes in for consideration. Alcoholic stimulants, used in moderation, often supply the place of starches and sugars that are difficult of digestion; and this is particularly true with those who are brain-workers.

A little stimulant to the aged brain-worker supplies the material for keeping up the animal heat without diverting the blood too much from the head; thus continued mental effort may be kept up for a considerable time with perfect safety. Elderly persons sleep less as they advance in years, and even at times they become affected by sleeplessness which is persistent. In such cases a light meal before retiring, with a glass of Tutonic Malt Extract, will draw the blood to the stomach, and favor natural sleep, while it is a valuable tissue builder.

FALLACIES REGARDING EATING.

Many fallacies regarding foods. and when to eat, are still entertained by the masses of the people, and a few of them will be briefly mentioned.

It is a fallacy to believe that man in health should live exclusively on a vegetable diet. It is true he may do so for a considerable length of time, but mixed animal and vegetable diet is more conducive to health and strength.

It is better to eat before going to bed than to go to bed hungry, as the stomach will digest the food during sleep more perfectly than at any other time, and besides a small quantity of food in the stomach, at bed-time, always draws a certain amount of blood from the brain, thus promoting natural sleep.

Many people find it impossible to eat certain kinds of food, as whenever they attempt it they have some unpleasant effects resulting therefrom.

In such cases, it is unwise to urge their eating them under any circumstances, as they are better able to judge for themselves from practical experience than anybody can judge for them. The old-fashioned beef-tea and the various extracts of beef on the market have little or no value as foods, as the processes by which they are prepared deprive them of their albumenoid substances, or so change their chemical composition as to render them valueless as tissue-builders.

The administra ion of food to sick persons by injection into the bowel we also believe to be a fallacy that has no foundation in fact. Foods thus introduced do not reach any tissue that takes up nutriment, and the only thing they can do is to remain there for a time and possibly cause irritation.

Condiments, as a rule, should be avoided, especially large quantities of pepper, mustard, and spicy sauces. These things, with salt, may be essential to give the proper flavor to food while cooking, but their free use on the food as eaten is often productive of much harm.

FOOD IN DYSPEPSIA.

Persons suffering from dyspepsia should abstain as far as possible from all foods containing much sugar and starch, as these substances undergo fermentation and cause an accumulation of gases in the stomach and bowels. Beef and mutton should be cooked rare so that the juice can be obtained. Game in any form should be avoided. Breasts of chicken or turkey should be eaten in preference to second joint. Pastry and farinaceous foods of all kinds must be abstained from. Care should be taken to thoroughly masticate the food, and drink should be avoided until complete mastication has been effected. Milk, especially skimmed milk, and eggs are wholesome. Scraped beef and animal broths may be used, while gluten bread should always be substituted for white flour bread.

FOOD IN BILIOUSNESS.

Persons who suffer from biliousness, without having any special accumulation of gases in the stomach, should eat fish, when it agrees with them, in preference to the meats. Vegetables, except potatoes, corn, and rice, may be eaten largely, and ripe fruits in their season, if they do not disagree with the stomach. Fat bacon is also a good article of food. Coffee as a rule is bad for most bilious persons, and experience will teach them that it should be avoided. A small quantity of fat meat is always preferable to the more solid portions. Eggs and milk should as a rule be avoided, although they may agree with some persons. Malt liquors of all kinds are especially objectionable, and, if any stimulant is taken, a light wine or a strong alcoholic stimulant is preferable.

FOOD IN NERVOUS PROSTRATION.

Persons suffering from nervous prostration due to mental overwork or long-continued sickness should have easily digested foods. Fish and fat of meats, especially bacon, will be found very serviceable. Good rich milk, or, better still, fresh cream should be taken freely, while the yolk of an egg beaten with a little sherry wine will serve a good purpose two or three times a day. Lettuce prepared with oil, as a salad, is also suggested, while stewed fruits are particularly serviceable. Good tenderloin steak, well chopped up before broiling and cooked rare, will be easily digested and impart strength. In these cases, however, a generous supply of vegetables will usually serve a better purpose than a meat diet.

FOOD IN ACUTE AND CHRONIC RHEUMATISM.

In these diseases the object is to avoid such articles of food as will tend to produce lithic acid. Fish, bread, potatoes, milk, sugar, butter, cheese, coffee, or cocoa in moderation, should comprise the diet of persons suffering from rheumatism or gout. The animal broths may also be found serviceable, and fruits in their season as a general rule are both agreeable and wholesome. The heavy meat diet should be avoided, as it contains most of the material that goes to form lithic acid. Fat bacon is the least objectionable of the meats.

FOOD IN DIABETES.

In diabetes all kinds of food that tend to produce sugar should be avoided, and hence we must exclude from the diet of a diabetic patient sugar in any form, beets, carrots, rice, all starchy puddings and pastry of all kinds, as well as fresh and preserved fruits. Milk, sweet wines, malt liquors and cider must also be avoided. The diet should consist of butcher's meat of all kinds, poultry, game, fish, animal broths, gluten bread, eggs, cheese, butter, cream, lettuce, celery, pickles if digestible, and radishes may be regularly used; while beans, cabbage, asparagus, and cauliflower may be eaten in moderation. Tea, coffee or cocoa may be taken, and also sour wines, brandy, and good whisky in moderation, if required.

FOOD IN BRIGHT'S DISEASE.

Beef, mutton and pork should as a rule be avoided or eaten with moderation. Celery, turnips, carrots, salads, raw and cooked fruits, may be taken when they are known to agree with the stomach. Soups or broths may at times be taken in moderation, while oatmeal or hominy porridge will often constitute a desirable breakfast. Cream in quantities, with plenty of butter and oil, may be taken freely. Milk is sometimes recommended, while the free use of grapes has been suggested as a cure for the disease. Alcoholic stimulants invariably do harm, and should be entirely avoided, except in extreme cases of nervous prostration.

FOOD IN CONSUMPTION.

In consumption fats and oils constitute a very important part of the diet. It should, therefore, be borne in mind that fat meats, especially bacon, rich cream, plenty of butter, with bread, cod liver oil, and preparations of malt, will do much to supply the excessive waste of the system. The fleshy portions of meat as a rule are not desirable and are imperfectly digested. Stimulants, especially Tutonic Malt Extract, can also be freely taken with good results. Milk and cream are usually more acceptable to young persons than the fats, and the yolk of eggs, with sherry wine, can also be used through the day with advantage. Persons suffering from consumption should eat at short intervals, but not too much at any one time.

DIET IN ACUTE DISEASES.

During the continuance of all acute diseases and inflammations the question of diet is an important one. Liquid nourishment as a general thing should be resorted to. Milk, brown bread, and a gruel made of oatmeal or barley will always be found beneficial. In fact the aim should be to give an abundant supply of heat-producing food. The acidulated drinks, with sugar, are also demanded, and wine or pure whisky or brandy will be found a valuable aid in carrying a patient through a critical period. The usual custom of giving beef tea during an acute sickness is a mistaken idea, as it contains little or no nourishment, and even if it did it would do little or no good.

FOOD IN CONVALESCENCE.

After the disease has spent itself and the patient is slowly recovering, such food as will build up the wasted tissues should be resorted to. Animal broths, beef juice, scraped beef, and beef steak, finely chopped before boiling and cooked rare, will be found valuable; and raw eggs beaten up with sherry wine may be used during the day with advantage. As the patient improves fish or chicken may be given for a change. Too much food, however, should not be given at one time, but the patient should be fed often so as to keep up a continuous supply of the nutritive material.

During convalescence from all acute or wasting diseases, Bovinine will be found of particular value, as it contains all the elements of beef in the most coneentrated form. It should be given at short intervals, and continued till the patient regains his strength.

In conclusion we would protest against the too common practice of urging people to take quantities of food when they have no inclination to do so. In such cases food will do harm instead of good, for as soon as the system is in condition to require food it will be demanded.

CHAPTER XVII.

Antidotes for Poisons.

For Opium— Strychnine— Arsenic— Lead—Aconite— Belladonna— Carbolic Acid— Chloroform — Coal Gas — Illuminating Gas — Oxalic Acid— Gelsemium— Chloral— Poisonous Mushrooms.

Poisoning by accident or design is of such frequent occurrence that a knowledge of the symptoms and antidotes of the more common forms of poisoning is of importance in every household. While we indicate the emergency treatment for such cases, it must be borne in mind that a physician should always be summoned as soon as possible, as many complications are likely to arise that require both judgment and scientific knowledge.

OPIUM.

Opium, in some of its numerous forms, is frequently taken in poisonous doses. The symptoms are drowsiness, stupor, pulse quick at first but soon becomes slow and full, slow and difficult breathing, paleness of the skin, cold clammy perspiration, and contracted pupils; and after a time a profound coma comes on.

Treatment.—An emetic should be given to unload the stomach. For this purpose a teaspoonful of ground mustard seed in a teacupful of warm water will usually act promptly, and is generally at hand. The patient must be kept awake by slapping, pinching and forcing him to walk in the open air. He should be made to drink freely of strong black coffee, and if the stupor increases strong ammonia should be held under the nostrils. If he can swallow, from two to five-drop doses of belladonna should be given every half hour till the pupils are dilated.

When the physician is called he should give hypodermic injections of atropine till the effect of the opium is counteracted.

Laudanum, paregoric, Godfrey's cordial, most all soothing syrups, and the various morphine salts, are all prepared from opium, and when any of these are taken the symptoms and treatment are the same as given when opium itself is used.

STRYCHNINE.

When an over-dose of strychnine or nux vomica is taken, the effect begins to be manifest in about fifteen or twenty minutes. The symptoms are a sense of suffocation, great difficulty of breathing, muscular trembling, twitching of the head, arms, and legs, and finally violent convulsions. These convulsions cause powerful muscular contractions and rigidity of the entire body, which may continue for a few minutes and then subside for a short interval, only to recur with greater severity with each paroxysm.

Treatment.—The spasms should be controlled by the inhalation of chloroform, and ten grains of camphor and one teaspoonful of chloroform should be given by the mouth, in a little whisky, at intervals of half an hour. When the spasms are once controlled twenty drops of tincture of gelsemium may be given every hour till the muscles are completely relaxed. When possible the treatment should be directed by a physician.

ARSENIC.

Arsenic is frequently employed as a poison, and is often swallowed by children in the form of rat-poison. When taken in large doses, faintness, nausea and vomiting, come on in from half an hour to one hour. An intense burning in the stomach is present, which continues to increase till severe purging takes place. Cramps of the abdomen and legs, constriction and dryness of the throat, intense thirst, feeble pulse, and cold and clammy skin are among the other symptoms present.

Treatment.—-The patient may drink freely of cold water, and two tablespoonfuls of dialyzed iron should be given every half hour. Friction and hot fomentations should be applied to the abdomen and extremities, and a quarter of a grain of morphine may be given in some cases, with advantage. This is best administered hypodermically by a physician.

LEAD.

Lead poisoning sometimes occurs from the metal being mixed with food or water, or by working in the metal. Painters, plumbers, and manufacturers of white lead, are liable to be thus poisoned.

This poisoning is of a chronic character, and it is first manifested by loss of appetite, poor digestion, constipation, colic, muscular paralysis, and the appearance of a bluish line on the margin of the gums.

Women who have used cosmetics containing lead often develop these symptoms without knowing how to account for them.

Treatment.—The person must discontinue using lead lotions, or working with metal in any form. The bowels should be kept regular by the use of our Home Liver Pills, and five grains of iodide of potassium should be taken three times a day.

ACONITE.

Aconite poisoning is speedily followed by tingling and numbness of the tongue, dizziness, loss of power, and numbness of the legs, severe abdominal pains vomiting and purging.

Treatment.—An emetic should be given as soon as possible. If the teaspoonful of mustard in a cupful of warm water fails to empty the stomach, thirty drops of fluid extract of ipecac should be given every twenty minutes till free vomiting is produced.

Friction of the extremities, hot applications to the abdomen, and the free use of whisky or brandy are also indicated. If the breathing fails artificial respiration and the inhalation of the fumes of nitrite of amyl should be resorted to.

BELLADONNA.

Dryness of the mouth and throat, nausea, vomiting, dizziness, dilated pupils, dullness of vision or double vision, mental excitement, delirium and convulsions are the symptoms of belladonna poisoning.

Treatment.—The first thing to do is to empty the stomach with an emetic. Then whisky or brandy should be given freely, and morphine one-fourth grain should be given by the mouth or hypodermically. Artificial respiration should also be kept up if the breathing begins to fail.

CARBOLIC ACID.

Carbolic acid has frequently been used of late with suicidal intent, and it is often swallowed by mistake. It acts as a caustic to the mucous surfaces of the mouth, throat and stomach, and causes a shock to the nervous system. Half a glassful of olive oil should be swallowed as soon as possible, and then the stomach should be emptied by an emetic. Hot applications to the extremities and hot brandy and water internally should then be used freely. The physician may often find it neces- sary to use a faradic current of electricity.

CHLOROFORM.

When too much chloroform has been inhaled, ammonia should be held under the nostrils and ar- tificial respiration should be resorted to. Nitrite of amyl should also be given by inhalation if the breathing is not speedily restored. In fact this remedy should always be on hand when chloroform is to be used for any purpose.

COAL GAS.

In poisoning from coal gas, the windows must be opened widely, ammonia should be inhaled, and artificial respiration should be employed. Hot mustard water should be applied to the feet and hands, and repeated shocks should be caused by alternately dashing hot and cold water on the face and chest. Electricity will also be found valuable in bringing about a reaction. Stimulants should be used freely as soon as the patient can swallow.

ILLUMINATION GAS.

The inhalation of illumination gas has become a common method of attempting suicide, and it is often turned on accidentally.

The same general treatment should be employed as is recommended for poisoning from coal gas.

OXALIC ACID.

Poisoning with oxalic acid occasions an intense and burning taste during swallowing, which extends into the stomach, causing a burning pain, vomiting, tenderness of abdomen, and drawing up of the legs.

The poison is antidoted by drinking freely of lime water, and afterward clearing the intestines with an ounce of castor oil.

GELSEMIUM.

Large doses of gelsemium causes drooping of the eyelids, double vision, fullness and pain in the head, and general muscular paralysis.

These conditions are readily overcome by the free use of whisky or brandy, and the inhalation of ammonia fumes.

In severe cases the inhalation of nitrite of amyl will promptly relieve the extreme depression.

CHLORAL.

An overdose of chloral always produces profound stupor with labored breathing.

The inhalation of nitrite of amyl is the quickest and surest antidote for chloral poisoning. When the patient revives somewhat heat and friction should be applied to the extremities and stimulant should be freely used.

POISONOUS MUSHROOMS.

Poisonous fungus growths are sometimes eaten in mistake for mushrooms. They occasion symptoms of intoxication, and a peculiar anomaly of vision, in which all objects look blue. Usually there is irritation of the stomach and bowels.

The first thing to be done is to empty the stomach with an emetic, and then move the bowels with an ounce of castor oil. Heat should be applied to the stomach and extremities, and stimulants should be given internally.

CHAPTER XVIII.

What to Do in Emergencies.

Burns and Scalds — Pistol Wounds — Bleeding from Wounds— Bleeding from the Nose — Bleeding from the Lungs—Fainting—Convulsions—Drowning–Accidents from Falls or Collisions.

Many emergencies arise in which prompt action is necessary either to save life or prevent much suffering. The suggestions here given are not claimed to cover the entire ground, but if studied they may often prove of value to the reader.

BURNS AND SCALDS.

The intense pain caused by burns or scalds is best relieved by bathing the part with a solution of one ounce of bicarbonate of soda to a pint of water. After this is poured on the burned surface pieces of old lint or muslin may be saturated in the solution and laid over the part, and then kept wet by pouring the solution over it till the burning pain is relieved. If the physician has not arrived by that time, cover the burn with sweet olive oil to exclude the air till the part can be permanently dressed by the doctor.

PISTOL WOUNDS.

If a person is wounded by a bullet from a pistol the first care is to see that any bleeding is arrested. If the ball has penetrated the chest or abdomen, the patient should be placed in a recumbent position, and all motion should be prevented till the physician arrives. If there is any indication of faintness or shock, an ounce of good whisky or brandy may be given.

BLEEDING FROM WOUNDS.

When severe bleeding occurs immediately after the receipt of a wound, a firm pressure with the fingers or thumbs, over the edge of the wound from which the blood comes will temporarily arrest its flow. If the blood flows with pulsating jets, it shows that an artery has been cut. In such cases pressure should be made between the wound and the heart, and the position of the pressure should be changed till the bleeding is controlled. Then tie a knot in the middle of a handkerchief, and place the knot over the point where the pressure of the fingers stopped the bleeding. Then tie the handker_ chief around the limb, place a stout stick between it and the skin, and then twist the stick till the knot presses deeply into the soft tissues, so as to press on the artery. Should this control the bleeding the patient is safe till the surgeon arrives

When the bleeding is slight, cold applications will often arrest it; or one handkerchief may be folded so as to form a compress, and another bound around the limb firmly so as to cause enough pressure to stop the bleeding.

In all cases of wounds where there is much bleeding, a surgeon should be summoned immediately, as the above directions are only intended for emergencies.

BLEEDING FROM THE NOSE.

Slight bleeding from the nose may often occur and last but a few moments. If it is severe, however, something should be done to stop it.

The first and simplest thing to do is to snuff cold water up the nostrils so as to allow it to pass down into the mouth. If this fails, ice should be applied to the back of the neck and to the bridge of the nose, and small pieces may be introduced into the nostrils. The finger or thumb may be pressed firmly against the under surface of the upper lip at its center, so as to press the lip against the nose, or a wad of paper or cotton may be crowded between the upper lip and the gum, and the lip then pressed against it from without.

If these means fail, a surgeon should be sent for to plug the nostrils from the mouth, or apply some astringent medicine.

BLEEDING FROM THE LUNGS.

When bleeding from the lungs takes place the blood is of a bright scarlet color, and has the appearance of froth, or foam. It is seldom present except in cases of consumption, and is usually a very unfavorable symptom.

The patient should be made to lie down at once, with the head and shoulders elevated. Common table salt should be given, in teaspoonful doses, every half hour till several doses are taken, and a hot mustard footbath should be given. The physieian should be sent for at once, but if the bleeding is not stopped before his arrival, ten drops of the oil of erigeron should be given in a tablespoonful of syrup, and repeated every fifteen or twenty minutes till four or five doses are taken. This remedy can be obtained in any drug store.

The patient should be kept quiet in bed for several days after an attack, and the diet should be of the most nourishing kind.

FAINTING.

When a person faints from any cause, he should be placed on the back, on a level surface, with the head lower than the body; the clothes should be loosened so as to leave the abdomen and chest free from pressure; ammonia or smelling salts should be held under the nostrils; and cold water may be dashed in the face to cause a slight shock. As soon as the patient can swallow, some good stimulant should be given; and quiet should be enforced till complete reaction has taken place.

CONVULSIONS, OR FITS.

In any case of convulsions, or fits, the first thing to be done is to take precautions against the patient hurting himself. If possible, a folded handkerchief should be crowded between the teeth, and the limbs should be held during each paroxysm.

In convulsions of infants a hot bath will often afford prompt relief.

The physician should be summoned immediately as experience alone can guide us in determining what treatment to follow in the different kinds of convulsions.

DROWNING.

When a person is asphyxiated from drowning, he should be laid upon his back and a person kneeling at his head should grasp the arms just below the elbows. The arms are then carried away from the sides, and then carried upward over the head, making a steady pull for a few seconds. Then carry the arms forward and down to the sides, at the same time making a firm, steady pressure on the sides of the lower ribs. These motions should be repeated fifteen or sixteen times per minute, till respiration is reestablished. It may often be necessary to keep up the movements for half an hour or longer before the suspended animation is restored. Ammonia may be held to the nostrils while these motions are being made.

As soon as there is an indication of returning animation, the wet clothes should be removed, friction and heat should be applied to the extremities, and stimulants should be given as soon as he can swallow.

ACCIDENTS FROM FALLS OR COLLISIONS.

If a person is stunned by a fall or a collision, or if any bones are broken, the first thing to do is to place him on his back and extend the arms and legs. Then the face may be bathed with cold water and ammonia held to the nostrils. If the condition is one of slight shock, consciousness will return in a short time; but if there is any injury to the brain or spinal cord the stupor may last a long time. Such patients should be removed to a hospital or their homes as soon as possible. If no ambulence can be had, a board, shutter, or door, can always be had to place the patient on, when he can easily be carried home. A surgeon should be summoned at once.

In cases of fractures or dislocations the proper treatment should be resorted to without delay, but in severe shock it is necessary to wait till reaction has been established before anything can be done.

CHAPTER XIX.

Our Home Medicines.

In offering to the public the following medicines prepared from the private prescriptions of the author, the Home Treatment Company feel confident that they are placing within reach of all remedies that will prove of great benefit to suffering humanity. They are the result of careful study and observation in an extensive private practice, extending over a period of thirty years; and a single trial will convince the most skeptical that they will do all that is claimed for them.

They are not patent medicines, or "*cure alls*," but each is prepared with special reference to the class of diseases for which it is recommended.

In most cases they have been prepared in PILL OR TABLET FORM, from the concentrated medicinal principles of plants and herbs, and are guaranteed pure and efficient. In this way we insure uniformity of dose, certainty of action convenience of administration at all times, and freedom from disagreeable tastes.

All medicines that will produce the desired effect must be more or less disagreeable to the taste when taken in liquid form, and our most valuable reme-

dies are intensely bitter.   It can therefore be laid
down as a rule that all tonics, malarial remedies,
kidney and liver medicines, dyspepsia cures, etc.,
that are pleasant to the taste in liquid form do not
have the strength necessary to produce proper
action.

To those who think they cannot swallow a pill
or tablet we would say, "Drop it in the mouth, behind the teeth and under the tongue, and immediately take one or two swallows of water, and the
pill is down before you know it."

HOME DYSPEPSIA PILLS.

*A specific for acute indigestion, chronic dyspepsia, heart-
burn, acid stomach, flatulency, bloating after eating, and wind colic.*

Home Dyspepsia Pills are specially compounded with the view of giving the requisite tone
and stimulus to the general system, and meeting
the requirements in the several disorders of digestion above named.

Among the symptoms indicating its use may be
mentioned a heavy or cutting pain in the stomach
soon after eating, a distended, full feeling of the
stomach and bowels, belching of wind and flatulence, a burning sensation in the stomach, heart-
burn, palpitation of the heart, oppression of breathing, pain under the ribs and shoulder-blades,

headache through the temples and eyes, dizziness, coated tongue, and constipation.

Many of these symptoms are absent, but some of them are always present in all cases of dyspepsia, while sometimes nausea and vomiting will occur before even temporary relief is obtained.

These symptoms are often attended with extreme despondency of spirits, when the patient looks on the dark side of everything, wishes he was dead, and even contemplates suicide.

Directions for Use.—One pill should be taken immediately after each meal, and the treatment should be continued till no discomfort is felt after eating. In long-standing cases it is best to begin with two pills at a dose and continue for ten or fourteen days. After that one pill will be suficient.

In all cases of acidity, flatulence, or feeling of bloating after eating, it is best to abstain from all foods containing starch and sugar. This would exclude potatoes, corn, rice, white bread, beets, sugar, sweetmeats, and pastry. The patient can still select from meats of all kinds, fish, raw oysters, beans, peas, lettuce, asparagus, tomatoes, ripe fruits in season, rye bread, and bread made from pure gluten flour. By adhering to this diet, acetous fermentation is prevented, and the remedies will restore the natural digestion more promptly.

If the bowels should be constipated, or the

tongue coated, our H o m e Liver Pills should be used at bed time.

Price, $1.00 per box.

HOME TONIC PILLS FOR WOMEN.

Specially compounded for the diseases and weaknesses peculiar to women.

H o m e Tonic Pills for Women are not only a valuable general tonic, but are also a special tonic for the womb and ovaries.

The great frequency of diseases of the womb, and the continued suffering to which they give rise, are due in part to the ignorance of women concerning themselves, and in part to their delicacy in consulting a physician. Every woman should read the chapter on " Diseases of Woman," and then by using this remedy most of their suffering will certainly be averted.

When a woman has pain in the small of the back, or at the lower end of the spine, a sensation of dragging and dull aching about the hips and thighs, a weight or fullness in the lower part of the abdomen, headache on the top or back of the head, with general languor and weakness, she may be certain that she is suffering from some disorder of the womb, while a frequent desire to urinate, and the presence of leucorrhea (whites) indicate more serious complications. These symptoms indicate the necessity for the use of this remedy. It can also be used with advantage during pregnancy and at "*the change of life.*"

Directions for Use.—One pill should be taken, fifteen or twenty minutes before each meal, at first; but if the symptoms are not greatly improved after ten days or two weeks, two pills can be taken before each meal.

When leucorrhea (whites) is present our H o m e Uterine Tablets should be used as directed on page 257.

Price, $1.00 per box of one hundred pills.

HOME MALARIAL PILLS.

A cure for chills, fever and ague, dumb ague, bilious fever, and all malarial fevers.

The H o m e Malarial Pills will effectually eradicate from the system all trace of the malarial poison, and when taken as directed will prevent any recurrence of these persistent and distressing complaints. It is guaranteed to contain no quinine, and hence does not produce the fullness of the head and ringing of the ears that follow the use of that drug.

When a person feels a sense of languor and depression, aching of the muscles and apparently of the bones, chilliness with alternate flashes of heat, a dull, heavy headache, and pain between and under the shoulder blades, with sometimes a decided chill followed by high fever and profuse perspiration, or a continued chilly feeling lasting for several hours. there can be no doubt of the malarial character of the disorder. When these symptoms recur about the same time every day, or every second or third day, the character of the disease is more fully assured.

Directions for Use.—One pill should be taken every three hours, while awake, for one week. Then omit the pill for about four days, after which it should be taken as before for three days more. In this way the treatment should be renewed for three days each week, omitting the other days, till a month has passed. This will insure a radical cure of the worst forms of malarial diseases.

As the action of the liver is óf great importance, our H o m e Liver Pills should be taken regularly during the treatment.

Price, $1.00 per box of one hundred pills.

Neurodine Tablet.

A specific for neuralgia, sciatica, nervous headache, toothache, hysterical spasms, insomnia, and nervous irritability.

Neurodine Tablets quiet and soothe all pain and nervous irritability, when the nervous system is primarily affected, by equalizing the circulation in the nerve centers.

It is not recommended for rheumatism and other painful inflammations, and should not be used in such cases. It is, however, a specific in all forms of neuralgia, toothache, nervous headache, hysterical spasms, and sleeplessness.

Directions for Use.—In sciatica, toothache, and all cases of neuralgia, take two tablets every half hour till relieved, or till six or eight tablets are taken. When pain is severe the patient should be in the recumbent position while taking the medicine and for a couple of hours afterward. In long standing cases one tablet should be taken after each meal, and before retiring one may be taken every half hour till five or six doses are taken.

For sleeplessness two tablets should be taken at bed-time, and one tablet every half hour afterward till sleep is produced.

For hysterical spasms one tablet should be taken, and repeated as above when spasms are present, but when the symptoms of extreme nervousness alone are present one tablet should be taken after each meal and two tablets at bed-time.

The tablet contains no narcotic, and as it acts only on the nerve centers, can be taken as directed with perfect safety.

When the dose is often repeated it will produce in very sensitive persons a relaxation of the muscles and a heaviness of the eyelids. These symptoms are of no consequence and are only mentioned to avoid uneasiness in the minds of those who might notice them. Keep quiet for a short time and such symptoms will soon disappear, as will also the pain.

Price, $1.00 per box of one hundred tablets.

HOME CHOLERA TABLETS.

For diarrhea, dysentery, cholera morbus, and cholera.

The H o m e Cholera Tablets are combined so as to promptly arrest the development of the intestinal disorders so commonly met with in the summer season. They are free from the disagreeable taste and tendency to nausea that is met with in the use of the liquid remedies so generally recommended. The tablets should be kept on hand by every family during the summer, and used according to directions as soon as any looseness of the bowels is noticed. In this way the more serious disorders, such as dysentery, cholera morbus, and cholera may be avoided.

Directions for Use. — For diarrhea one tablet should be taken every hour for three or four hours. This will usually relieve the worst cases, though sometimes five or six doses will be necessary.

For dysentery or cholera morbus two tablets should be taken at first, and then one tablet in half an hour. The one tablet may be given at intervals of half an hour for four or five times afterward, if necessary to control the bowels.

In all cases the medicine should be discontinued

as soon as relief is obtained, but can be renewed when a recurrence takes place.

For children between six and ten years of age, the tablets should be cut in two with a sharp knife, and one-half given not oftener than once an hour.

For children under six, and over three years of age, the tablet should be crushed into a powder, and one-fourth given at a dose a couple of times, with an hour's interval between the doses. It should not be given to children under three years of age.

During the continuance of these disorders it is best to avoid much food, as it is not digested and only aggravates the disease. Fluids should be abstained from as much as possible, excepting boiled milk in moderation. Starchy foods are preferable to any other, and in bad cases absolute rest is always a great help.

After the disease is controlled the bowels are usually constipated. To relieve this use our Home Liver Pills.

Price, $1.00 per box of one hundred tablets.

HOME LIVER PILLS.

A radical cure for constipation, biliousness, bilious and sick headache, colic, and torpid liver.

Our Home Liver Pills can always be taken with safety and with a certainty of producing the desired effect.

In all cases of constipation they will not only relieve the difficulty at the time, but will overcome it entirely.

Their use is indicated when the tongue is coated with a brown or whitish coating; when there is a dull pain under the lower ribs on the right side, extending around under the shoulder-blades; when there is a pain low down on the left side of the abdomen; when the eyes and skin look yellowish; when there are brown moth-spots on the face and other parts of the body; and when there is a pain through the eyes, or severe headache with sickness of the stomach.

Directions for Use.—As these pills are made so as to be given in small doses, no person should take more than one pill on going to bed. This can be continued every night till the bowels move freely more than once a day, after which one pill should be taken every second or third night, till the tongue is clear and all pain relieved.

In cases where the bowels do not move freely after the third night, two pills may be taken at bed-time till the desired effect is produced; then continue with one pill as required.

In this way an efficient and pleasant action can be secured, without any of the harsh effects of strong cathartics.

In some cases even three pills may be required, but in all cases only one should be taken at a dose to begin with.

Price, 25 cents per box of twenty-five pills; $1.00 per box of one hundred and twenty-five pills.

HOME RHEUMATIC PILLS.

A certain cure for rheumatism, gout, lumbago, and pains in muscles and joints.

The H o m e Rheumatic Pills will be found the most valuable and certain cure for all forms of rheumatism and gout that has yet been offered to the public. They are compounded with special reference to the causes of these diseases, and will not only relieve them but radically remove the cause.

Remember that neuralgia and sciatica belong to another class of diseases, and cannot be relieved by a rheumatic remedy.

Directions for Use.—Take one pill after each meal and at bed-time. Continue the treatment till the pain is entirely relieved.

If the bowels are constipated they should be kept loose by using our H o m e Liver Pills.

Price, $1.00 per box of one hundred pills.

HOME NERVE TONIC PILLS.

A radical cure for nervous debility, general prostration, loss of manhood, impotence, and spermatorrhea.

The Home Nerve Tonic Pills is the only remedy that can be used with the certainty of producing imme-

diate beneficial results in the conditions for which
they are recommended.

In all cases of general or nervous debility, impotence, and spermatorrhea, they act as a powerful
special tonic, and can truly be called a specific.

Such cases are not incurable, as has been so
often asserted. These pills will permanently restore
lost vigor in all cases that do not require special
surgical treatment.

Directions for Use.—One pill should be taken
fifteen or twenty minutes after each meal, and
should be continued for two or three months. In
most cases, however, a decided improvement is
manifested before the first box is taken. A tepid
sponge bath every morning, followed by twenty
minutes' rubbing with a coarse towel, will prove of
great advantage in conjunction with the pills.

If the bowels should be constipated, and the
tongue coated, our H o m e Liver Pills should be
used.

Price, $1.50 per box of one hundred pills.

HOME ALTERATIVE PILLS.

*A never-failing blood purifier in scrofula, salt rheum,
eczema, ring worm, syphilis, skin eruptions, and
all disorders of the blood.*

The Home Alterative Pills are compounded
with the special view of taking the place of the
large and disagreeable doses of liquid "Blood

Purifier" that people have so long been persuaded to use.

They are applicable to all conditions of the blood that give rise to skin eruptions, glandular swellings, ulcerations, boils, pimples, scabs, etc.

They contain neither mercury nor potash, and instead of reducing the system they builds up and enrich the blood, throwing off the poison and restoring health.

Directions for Use.—One pill should be taken after each meal and at bed-time, and continued with regularity till all symptoms of the disease disappear. In old cases this treatment should be persistently followed for three or four months.

When a person has been exposed to any specific poison, like syphilis, a prompt use of this remedy will prevent it from getting into the blood.

Price, $1.50 per box of one hundred pills.

HOME KIDNEY PILLS.

A never-failing remedy in congestion and inflammation of the kidneys, Bright's disease, gravel, irritation and inflammation of the bladder, suppression of urine, and all disorders of the kidneys and bladder, and to reduce dropsical swellings.

Diseases of the kidneys are the most common that affect mankind, and when neglected are the most liable to become chronic and terminate fatally. These disorders are fully described in Chapter IX, page 130, of this manual; and when any of the symptoms therein described are recognized, no time should be lost in having the urine analyzed.

Our H o m e Kidney Pills, when used according to directions, will always act promptly on the kidneys, increasing the flow of urine, relieving pains in the back, allaying irritation of the bladder, and a frequent desire to urinate, and reducing dropsical conditions caused by Bright's disease.

They also act powerfully in dissolving gravel in the kidneys and bladder, thus preventing the formation of stone in the bladder.

One pill should be taken every three hours; but in cases of dropsy and when the flow of urine is very scanty, two pills should be taken every three hours.

These pills should not be taken for diabetes.

Price, $1.50 per box of one hundred pills.

HOME SPECIFIC PILLS AND TABLETS.

A specific in gonorrhea, gleet, and inflammation of the prostate gland.

H o m e Specific Pills, in conjunction with Home Specific Tablets, will cure the worst cases of gonorrhea, in from three to six days, if used in time, and according to directions.

One pill should be taken every three hours; and one tablet should be dissolved in two tablespoonfuls of water and used as an injection, after urinating, and repeated three or four times a day.

In long standing cases of gleet or inflammation of the prostate gland Specific Tablet No. 2 should be used for the injection, and two of our H o m e Specific Pills should be taken at a dose.

The H o m e Specific Pills and Tablets, with syringe, securely packed, sent by mail for $3.00.

HOME EYE TABLETS.

H o m e Eye Tablets will promptly cure inflammation of the eyes, weak eyes, and recent cases of granulated eyelids.

One tablet should be dissolved in an eyebath full of tepid water, and the eye bathed three or four times a day. Directions for using eyebath aecompanics the tablets.

Price, per box of fifty tablets and eyebath, $1.00,

HOME UTERINE TABLETS.

These tablets are prepared especially for the home treatment of leucorrhea (whites), inflammation of the womb and vagina, and the several forms of displacement of the womb. They have been used by the author in an extended practice of thirty years, and are guaranteed to cure seventy-five per cent. of the diseases and weaknesses peculiar to women.

When used in connection with the H o m e Tonic Pills for Women, the most satisfactory results are obtained; and in the majority of cases they do away with the necessity of consulting a physician and submitting to local examinations.

These tablets are intended for the local treat-ment of diseases of the womb and vagina, and full directions for their use accompanies each box.

Price, $1.00 per box, and this will save twelve visits to a physician.

HOME WORM LOZENGES.

The Home Worm Lozenges are an efficient and harmless remedy in all cases of stomach worms. When worms are suspected the child should be kept on as little food as possible during the afternoon, and to a child under two years of age two of the lozenges should be given in the evening. If the bowels do not move freely before ten o'clock, a dose of castor oil should be given before noon-time, and if worms are present they are sure to come away before night. Children over two years of age may take one lozenge every hour till four or five are taken, and it is always best to give the oil in the morning. If no worms are seen in the passages, it is a sure indication that none were present.

Price, 50 cents per box.

HOME COUGH LOZENGES.

In all cases of coughs and colds, when the throat is irritated and the cough annoying, relief is speedily obtained and expectoration promoted by the free use of the H o m e Cough Lozenges. They will also be found of great value in cases of sore throat; and in the severer coughs of bronchitis and consumption they will soothe and quiet the cough without producing any unpleasant symptoms.

Directions for Use.—A lozenge should be taken into the mouth and allowed to dissolve, and the saliva slowly swallowed as it accumulates. Five or six may be thus used in succession, and in severe cases their use can be continued till the irritation is relieved. They can be repeated in the same way at intervals of an hour or two.

They can be used with even young children, but to children under three years of age only one should be given every hour at first, and after three or four are taken the interval should be extended to two hours.

They can be used with great benefit in all cases where nauseating syrup and cough mixtures were formerly given.

Price, 50 cents per box.

HOME OINTMENT.

For burns, scalds, eczema, acne, cuts, etc.

H o m e Ointment should find a place in every household. It is composed of the best-known antiseptics, and will speedily cure all skin eruptions, burns, scalds, and wounds.

Full directions for use accompanies each box.

. Price, 50 cents a box.

HOME PILE OINTMENT.

H o m e Pile Ointment is a specific for all cases of recent piles, and will palliate even severe cases, till an operation can be performed. It relieves the pain, itching, and burning, and rapidly contracts the protruding mass.

It must be applied well up the bowel, with the finger two or three times a day.

Price, $1.00 per box.

HOME CORN SALVE.

H o m e Corn Salve will permanently remove corns and calluses in three or four days, and when used according to directions will prevent their recurrence.

Price, 25 cents per box.

THE   HOME   INHALER.

A radical cure for catarrh, and the best-known method of treating bronchitis, consumption, asthma, and hay fever, that has yet been offered to the public.

The H o m e Inhaler does not produce a spray, but a medicated air that can be forced into every minute crevice of the air passages of the nose and inhaled to the air cells of the lungs. Thus a medicated air is brought in direct contact with the diseased parts and a healthy action is at once set up.

Full directions for use accompany each instrument.

Inhalent No. 1 is prepared specially for the treatment of catarrh, sore throat, and irritation of the bronchial tubes.

Inhalent No. 2 is used in cases of hay fever, influenza, and consumption.

Our Asthma Inhalation is to be used with the same instrument in all cases of genuine asthma or spasmodic breathing due to heart troubles or any nervous disorder.

The instrument is put up in a substantial box with Inhalent No. 1 or 2, as desired, and sent to any address, by express prepaid, for $3.00

The asthma cure with the Inhaler will be sent for the same price.

HOME ASTHMA INHALATION.

Our Home Asthma Inhalation, when used in our Vitakure Inhaler, will relieve the paroxysms of asthma more promptly than any other remedy; and when used several times a day it will prevent their recurrence for long periods of time.

The use of this Inhalation and the observance of the general treatment recommended on pages 91 and 92 of this manual will prove a blessing to asthma sufferers.

Price of Inhaler and Asthma Inhalation $3.00.

THE EARTH-MAGNETO ELECTRIC BATTERY.

The value of Electricity as one of the forces of nature in the treatment of disease, has long been recognized by the medical profession, but the various batteries devised for the purpose have failed to meet the requirements and could not be trusted to laymen without danger.

The Earth-Magneto Battery is the most recent and most wonderful scientific discovery of the age, as it generates an electrical force, which can be applied without shock or burning of the skin, which possesses more curative power than any electric current heretofore used.

Wherever electricity is recommended in this book, this is the form of current that should be employed. It is especially designed for home use, and when used according to directions the body can be charged with electric force without any possibility of injury.

The Earth-Magneto combines the Static Magnetic and Galvanic forms of Electricity in such form that it can be used on the most sensitive person, without shock, or unp'easant sensation, and if necessary, it can be applied at bed time and left on all night. It is specially applicable in nervous prostration, nervous headache, rheumatism, lumbago, neuralgia, and defective circulation from any cause. Full directions aecompany each battery. This battery is manufactured by the Earth-Magneto Medical Battery Co., 19 Union Square, New York.

INDEX.

Abscess of the Ear 194
Absence of Conjugal Desire 175
        Menstruation 165
Accidents from Falls or Collisions 242
Accumulation of Wax 193
Acne...................................151
Acute Bronchitis......................... 87
        Diseases, Diet in.....................227
        Indigestion 18
        Nasal Catarrh 92
Adult Life, Food for.......................219
Amaurosis................................189
Angina Pectoris...........................128
Antidotes for Poisons......................229
Anus, Fissure of the.......................199
        Fistula of the.......................198
Asthma.................................. 90
        Inhalation 261
Astigmatism..............................182
Balanitis 144
Barbers Itch.............................162
Barrenness 176
Battery, Electric 262
Bed Sores 152
Biliousness 24
        Food in............................242
Bladder, Inflammation of the 138

Bladder, Stone in the........................138
Bleeding from the Nose.......................239
            Lungs 240
            Womb......................238
Blood Diseases, Specific...................... 76
Boils.......................................153
Bones, Diseases of 201
Bowed Legs 206
Bright's Disease............................132
            Food in....................226
Bronchitis, Acute............................ 87
            Chronic 88
Burns and Scalds........ ....162, 237
Caries........ 154
Care of the Eyes............................179
            Ears.......................191
Carbuncles 154
Cataract...................................188
Catarrh, Acute Nasal........................ 92
            Chronic....................102
            Of the Stomach............. 22
Cancers.............................176, 209
Chilblains 155
Chicken Pox................................ 46
Cholera.................................... 49
            Infantum................... 30
            Morbus..................... 27
            Tablets....................250
Chronic Bronchitis 88
            Catarrh....................102
            Diarrhea 26
            Dyspepsia.................. 19
Clap......................................142
Club Foot..................................207
Constipation, Habitual...................... 33
Consumption................................ 83
            Food in....................227

Conjunctivitis.................................186
Congestion of the Kidneys....................131
Conjugal Desire, Absence of.................175
Cornea, Ulceration of the...................187
        Opacity of the.......................187
Cough Lozenges 258
Convulsions..........................112, 241
        Food in.............................228
Cross-Eye 185
Croup....................................... 97
        Membranous.......................... 98
        Spasmodic........................... 98
Dandruff 156
Deafness 195
Defects of Vision...........................180
Defective Nutrition, Diseases of............ 64
Diabetes.................................... 71
        Food in.............................226
Diarrhea.................................... 25
        Chronic............................. 26
Diet in Acute Diseases......................227
Digestion, Organs of 13
Diphtheria.................................. 52
Diseases of the Bones 201
        Heart..............................123
        Joints 203
        Lids................................183
        Lungs and Air Passages....... 82
        Nervous System................106
Diseases and Injuries of the Skin.......... 151
Diseases of Defective Nutrition............. 64
Diseases of Women 164
Diseases, Urinary...........................130
Dislocations 203
Displacements of the Womb 171
Drowning...................................244
Drooping of the Lids 182

Dysentery 28
Dyspepsia, Chronic.......................... 19
        Food in............................223
        Pills.............................244
Ear, Abscess of the.........................194
    Polypus of the..........................194
    Care of the.............................191
Eating, Fallacies Regarding 222
Eczema......................................157
Emergencies, What to do in..................237
Enlargement of the Heart....................127
Epilepsy....................................113
Erysipelas.................................. 49
Eyes, Care of the...........................179
        Weeping, or Watery...................185
Eye and its Disorders.......................178
        Tablets..............................257
Fainting....................................240
Fallacies Regarding Eating..................222
Falling Out of Hair.........................156
Fatty Degeneration of the Heart.............127
Feeding, Infant.............................216
Fever, Bilious.............................. 40
    Intermittent............................ 39
    Hay.................................... 55
    Scarlet................................ 47
    Typhoid 61
Fissure of the Anus 199
Fistula of the Anus.........................198
Fits 241
Flesh Worms 151
Food for Adult Life.........................219
Food in Biliousness.........................224
    Bright's Disease.......................226
    Consumption 227
    Convalescence 228
    Diabetes 226

Food in Dyspepsia.............................223
      Health and Disease...................212
      Nervous Prostration................225
      Old Age............................221
      Rheumatism.........................225
Fractures....................................202
Freckles.....................................158
Germ Diseases, Specific........................ 43
Glanders 80
Glaucoma.,..................................189
Gleet..143
Gonorrhea...................................142
Gout 69
Granulated Lids.............................186
Gravel......................................134
Hair, Falling Out of........................156
Habitual Constipation........................ 33
Hay Fever.................................... 55
Headache....................................107
      Plethoric 108
      Rheumatic..........................108
      Sick...............................108
Heat, Prickley..............................159
Heart, Disease of the.......................123
      Enlargement........................127
      Fatty Degeneration of the...........127
Heart, Rheumatism of the....................123
      Palpitation of the.................124
Health, How to Preserve 16
Hernia 200
Hiccough....................................117
Hives 158
How to Preserve Health...................... 16
      Corn Salve.........................260
      Cough Lozenges.....................258
Hydrocele...................................146
Hypermetropia...............................181
Hysteria 115, 174
Indigestion, Acute 18

Infant Feeding......................216
Inflammation of the Bladder...................138
        Larynx..................100
        Kidneys..................131
        Vulva...................169
        Womb ....170 .
Influenza, Epidemic....................... 54
Ingrown Toe Nails...........................201
Impotence.........................149
Intestinal Worms..................... 34
Involuntary Escape of Urine..................139
Iritis.........................188
Irritation, Spinal.......................111
Itch.........................161
    Barbers......................162
Jaundice......................... 25
Joints, Diseases of the....................203
Kidneys, Congestion of the 131
Kidney Pills.........................255
Knock Knee......................... 206
Laceration of the Neck of the Womb...........172
        Perineum...................176
La Grippe......................... 54
Larynx, Inflammation of the..................100
Leucorrhea 173
Lids, Diseases of the 183
    Granulated.........................186
Liver Pills.........................251
Loss of Voice 100
Lungs, Bleeding from......................240
Malarial Diseases 38
    Fevers......................... 39
    Pills.........................247
Malformation and Injuries of the Ear..........193
Measles 46
Men, Special Diseases of.....................141
Menstruation, Absence of...................165

Menstruation, Painful.........................166
     Profuse........................167
Mumps.. 59
Myopia, or Near Sight........................181
Nasal Catarrh, Acute........................ 92
Near Sight...................................181
Neck of the Womb, Laceration of.............172
Nervous Prostration, Food in 225
   System, Diseases of the............106
Neuralgia....................................119
Neurodine Tablets 248
Nettle Rash 158
Nose, Bleeding from the.....................239
  Ulceration of the...................... 94
Ointment....................................259
Old Age, Food in 221
Old Sight...................................181
Opacity of the Cornea 187
Organs of Digestion........................ 13
Palpitations of the Heart...................124
Painful Menstruation........................166
Paraphimosis................................145
Paralysis...................................121
Perineum, Laceration of.....................174
Phymosis....................................144
Pile Ointment...............................260
Piles 196
Pistol Wounds 238
Pleurisy....................................104
Pneumonia...................................104
Poisons, Antidotes for......................229
Poisoning, Antidotes for Aconite............232
      Arsenic.............231
      Belladonna..........233
      Carbolic Acid 223
      Chloroform..........234
      Chloral 235

Poisoning. Antidotes for Coal Gas............234
                            Gelsemium...........235
                            Illuminating Gas......234
                            Lead................232
                            Opium...............229
                            Oxalic Acid.........235
                            Poisonous Mushrooms 236
                            Strychnine...........230
Polypus of the Ear 194
Presbyopia, or Old Sight......................181
Prickley Heat................................159
Profuse Menstruation 167
Quinsy.... 95
Retention of Urine............................136
Rheumatic Pills.............................253
Rheumatism.................................. 64
            Food in........................225
            Of the Heart....................125
Rickets.................................... 71
Ring Worm.................................159
Rupture...................................200
Salt Rheum.................................160
Sarsaparilla Pills. 154
Scarlet Fever............................. 47
Scalds. 162
Scrofula.................................. 74
Sea Sickness...............................118
Self-abuse 147
Skin, Diseases and Injuries of................151
Small-Pox............................... 44
Sore Throat.............................. 94
Special Diseases of Men 141
Specific Blood Diseases. 76
            Germ Diseases.................. 43
            Pills and Tablets...............256
Spermatorrhea.............................148
Spectacles, The Use of......................182

Spinal Deformities...........................205
    Irritation...............................111
Sprains......................................202
Stomach, Catarrh of the 22
Stone in the Bladder.........................138
Sterility....................................176
Stricture....................................145
Stys...184
St. Vitus Dance 114
Summer Complaint............................. 30
Surgical Diseases and Accidents..............196
Swelled Testicle.............................146
Syphilis..................................... 76
The Ear and its Disorders 190
Throat, Sore................................. 94
Testicle, Swelled............................146
Toe Nails, Ingrown 201
Tonic Pills for Women........................246
Torpid Liver................................. 24
Tumors.............................. ....176, 208
Typhoid Fever................................ 61
Ulcers.......................................207
Ulceration of the Cornea.....................187
    Nose..................................... 94
    Womb 171
Urine, Retention of..........................136
Uterine Tablets..............................257
Urine, Involuntary Escape of.................139
Urinary Diseases.............................130
Use of Spectacles............................182
Varicose Veins...............................200
Varicocele...................................147
Vertigo......................................111
Vision, Defects of...........................280
H o m e Cholera Pills........................250

HOME Dyspepsia Pills....................244
        Eye Tablets. 257
        Electric Battery 261
        Family Medicines...................243
        Inhaler...............................261
        Kidney Pills 255
        Liver Pills 251
        Malarial Pills.......................247
        Nerve Pills..........................253
        Ointment............................259
        Pile Ointment.......................260
        Rheumatic Pills. 253
        Alterative Pills.................. ...254
        Specific Pills and Tablets.............256
        Tonic Pills for Women. 246
        Uterine Tablets.....................257
        Worm Lozenges. 258
Voice, Loss of..............................100
Vulva.....................................167
        Inflammation of the..................167
Warts...... 161
Wax, Accumulation of.....................193
Weeping, or Watery Eyes..................185
What to Do in Emergencies...............237
Whooping Cough......................... 58
Womb, Displacements of the..............172
        Inflammation of the..................170
        Ulceration of the....................171
Women, Diseases of......................164
Worm, Ring. 159
        Lozenges..........................258
Worms, Intestinal........................ 34
        Round............................ 35
        Tape............................. 36
        Thread........................... 35
Wounds, Bleeding from 238
        Pistol,,,,,,,,,,,,,,,,,,,,,,,,,,,,,,,238

The remedies recommended in this book are carefully [pre]pared from formulas of a well-known physician and surg[eon] who has used them in his active practice for 30 years. They [are] not "PATENT MEDICINES NOR CURE-ALLS," but SPECIAL medic[ines] adapted to the scientific treatment of each class of diseases.

These remedies are in the form of pills and tablets, and [are] not unpleasant to the taste.

Dr. Gunn's Home Liver Pill.—*A radical cure for Constipa[tion], Biliousness, Bilious and Sick Headache, Colic and Torpid L[iver].* (These pills are the most perfect and satisfactory liver [pill] ever offered to the public. They have received the indo[rse]ments of many physicians, and of thousands of persons [who] have used them.) One pill is a dose. 25 for 25 cents; [50] or $1.00.

Dr. Gunn's Home Dyspepsia Pill.—A specific for acute Indi[ges]tion, Chronic Dyspepsia, Heartburn, Acid Stomach, Fl[atu]lancy, Bloating after eating, and Wind Colic. 50 cents [and] $1.00 per box.

Dr. Gunn's Home Malarial Pill.—A cure for Chills, Fever [and] Ague, Dumb Ague, Bilious Fever and all Malarial Fev[ers]. 50 cents and $1.00 per box.

Dr. Gunn's Home Rheumatic Pill.—A certain cure for Rheu[ma]tism, Gout, Lumbago, and pains in the muscles and jo[ints]. 50 cents and $1.00 per box.

Dr. Gunn's Neurodine Tablet.—A specific for Neuralgia, Scia[tica] Nervous Headache, Toothache, Hysterical Spasms, Sl[eep]lessness, and Nervous Irritability. 50 cents and $1.00 [per] box.

Dr. Gunn's Home Alterative Pill.—A never-failing blood pur[ifier] in Scrofula, Salt Rheum, Eczema, Ringworm, Syphilis, S[kin] eruptions, Pimples on the face and all disorders of [the] blood. 50 cents and $1.00 per box.

Dr. Gunn's Home Diuretic Pill.—A reliable remedy in conges[tion] and inflammation of the Bladder, Suppression of Ur[ine] and all disorders of the Kidneys and Bladder, and to red[uce] Dropsical swellings. 50 cents and $1.00 per box.

Dr. Gunn's Home Cholera Pill.—For Diarrhœa, Dysentery, C[hol]era Morbus and Cholera. 50 cents and $1.00 per box.

Dr. Gunn's Home Cough Lozenge.—A pleasant and efficaci[ous] remedy for Coughs, Colds, Sore Throat, and Bronch[itis]. 25 and 50 cents per box.

Dr. Gunn's Home Worm Lozenge.—A radical cure in all cas[ ] stomach worms. Palatable to the taste and certain [ ] result. 25 cents per box.

Dr. Gunn's Home Nerve Tonic Pill.—A radical cure for Ner[ ] Debility, General Prostration. Loss of Manhood. Impot[ ] and Spermatorrhœa or Nocturnal emissions. $1.50 per [ ]

[D]r. Gunn's Home Tonic Pill for Women.—This is a general [ ] as well as a special tonic for the Womb and Ovaries. [ ] the woman's friend, and when used in connection with [ ] HOME SUPPOSITORIES, will cure all cases of female weak[ ] $1.00 per box.

Dr. Gunn's Home Supposatories for Women.—These Supposat[ ] are prepared for the local treatment of diseases of the W[ ] and Vagina. With them every woman can cure herse[ ] all female disorders, without going to a physician for t[ ] ment. $1.00 per box.

N. B.—All boxes sold for $1.00 contain 100 pills, or [ ] cent per dose.

By reading the HOME DOCTOR carefully, you may [ ] physicians' fees.

By sending for HOME TREATMENT REMEDIES you will se[ ] FRESHLY prepared medicines, carefully compounded from [ ] drugs (not stale goods from druggists' shelves) AT WHOLE[ ] RATES. WHY? Because we have none of the expenses, pr[ ] extensive advertising, transportation, etc., etc., of middle[ ] which is enormous and is all paid for by the consumer. [ ] FORWARD OUR REMEDIES DIRECT TO THE PURCHASER BY M[ ] and therefore our patrons will receive the benefit of drug[ ] profits and get the most reliable remedies at the lowest rate[ ]

HOME TREATMENT REMEDIES are put up in plain pack[ ] with no indication of their contents. A question blank i[ ] closed with every HOME DOCTOR. If it is carefully fille[ ] and sent to us, our physicians will diagnose and give a[ ] without charge. Special question blanks, for diseases of [ ] and women will be sent on application. Correspondence or [ ] physical ailment will receive prompt attention. ALL COMM[ ] CATIONS ARE CONFIDENTIAL.

Our physicians can be consulted in all complicated [ ] and the best advice on all chronic and surgical diseases c[ ] relied on.

...1896...

hy the Waverley Succeeds

in presenting our '96 catalogue, which will be ready by January, we will endeavor to show in a clear, comprehensive manner, "Why the Waverley Succeeds." Our statements will be couched in plain every-day language that any child may read and understand. The catalogue will be fully illustrated, showing the various departments of our plant, with the workmen engaged in their different occupations, enabling our readers to grasp more readily the full meaning of our story. This advertisement i intended as a mere forerunner of the catalogu to come, and whether you buy a machine before hand or not, do not fail to get a copy of ou regular catalogue, as we are sure it will prov interesting to every wheelman. . . . .

diana Bicycle Co.

Factory, Indianapolis, Ind.

Street and B'way,
N. Y. City.

339 Broadwa
N. Y. City,

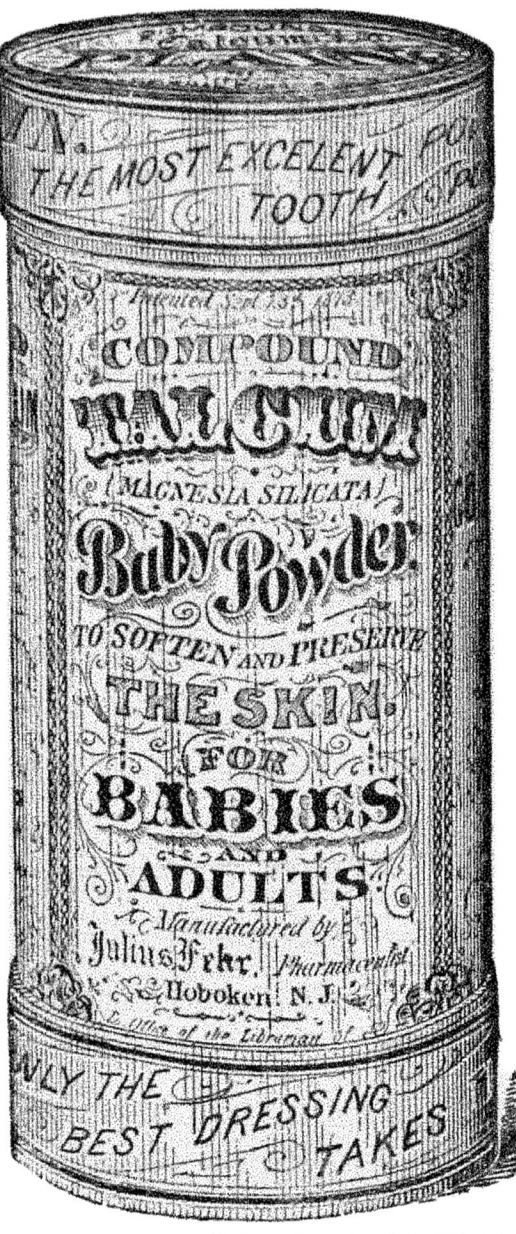

A · HOME · ORCHESTR

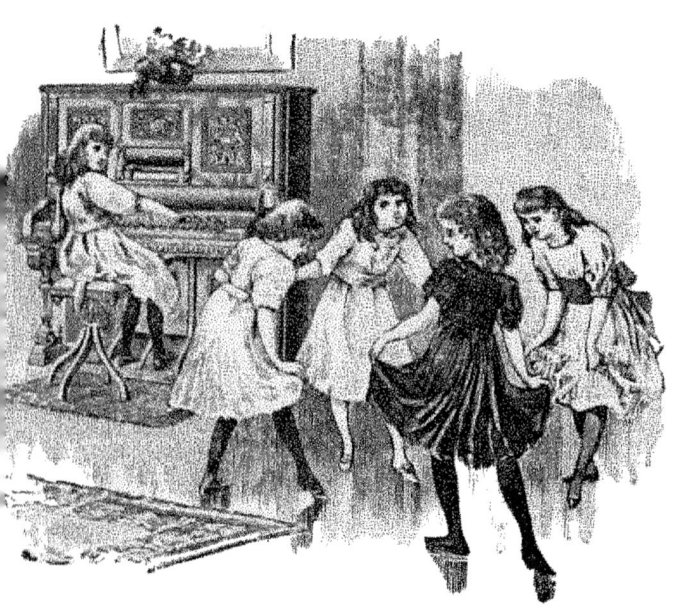